fight fatigue
the
7-day
diet
plan

carolyn humphries

D1432203

foulsham
LONDON • NEW YORK • TORONTO • SYDNEY

foulsham

The Publishing House, Bennetts Close, Cippenham,
Slough, Berkshire, SL1 5AP, England

ISBN 0-572-03094-0

Copyright © 2005 W. Foulsham & Co. Ltd

Cover photograph by Laurie Evans

A CIP record for this book is available from the British Library

Neither the editors of W. Foulsham & Co. Ltd nor the author nor
the publisher take responsibility for any possible consequences
from any treatment, procedure, test, exercise, action or
application of medication or preparation by any person reading
or following the information in this book. The publication of this
book does not constitute the practice of medicine, and this book
does not attempt to replace any diet or instructions from your
doctor. The author and publisher advise the reader to check with
a doctor before administering any medication or undertaking any
course of treatment or exercise.

Printed in Great Britain by Creative Print and Design (Wales), Ebbw Vale

CONTENTS

INTRODUCTION

Are you feeling tired, lethargic and listless every day? Do you have trouble concentrating for lengthy periods and just don't seem to have the energy you used to?

Fatigue is a common complaint. Nearly a third of adults in the UK and around half of those in the US suffer from chronic sleepiness. Obviously that number includes people with actual illnesses, such as post-viral fatigue syndrome, but for many of us it is a constant problem even when we are relatively well. Most people blame it on stress or the pace of modern life and, of course, these can be contributing factors, but for many people their diet is the main culprit. Did you know, for instance, that if you eat a huge, greasy breakfast, such as bacon, eggs, fried bread and sausages, you'll feel fabulously full but sluggish and sleepy and find it hard to concentrate all morning? If you pile into a pub lunch – pie and chips, for example, washed down with a cool lager – as likely as not, you'll be dragging yourself around most of the afternoon too! And I bet you didn't know that drinking a triple espresso won't keep you stimulated: it'll just give you a quick boost, then sap your energy, leading to restlessness, anxiety and fatigue.

Don't worry, this book is not about eating cranky health foods and never letting alcohol pass your lips again. But it will show you how simply including the right foods in your diet will keep you bright, alert and fit. As well as general healthy eating and lifestyle tips to point you in the right direction, there's a seven-day meal plan to set you off on the right road and loads of ideas for breakfasts, lunches, dinners and snacks to keep you firing on all cylinders all the time.

Even better, all my recipes are really easy to make, quick to prepare and taste absolutely superb. So awaken your taste buds as well as your body with this fatigue-fighting diet plan and see just how alive you start to feel!

FATIGUE AND HOW TO FIGHT IT

Feeling permanently tired affects everything you do and can make life miserable. It's a very common problem, but it's not always easy to pinpoint exactly what is causing it because there is a huge number of possible contributing factors. These may be anything from straightforward lack of sleep – caused by such things as overwork, too many late nights or the arrival of a new baby – to an underlying illness that has not been diagnosed. It is important, therefore, that you should take care to ensure that you establish the root of your own problems before you embark on any treatment.

WHAT CAUSES CHRONIC TIREDNESS?

In this section you'll find a list of possible causes. This is for information only and does not constitute an attempt to define your specific problem. I recommend that you go to your doctor if you are suffering from permanent tiredness. In many cases, a change of diet can go a long way to putting things right, but your doctor may wish to prescribe something that will help. He or she will also be able to check that there is nothing more serious wrong with you.

Anaemia
One of the most common causes of chronic tiredness is anaemia. This happens when the blood doesn't have enough red blood cells to carry oxygen round the body efficiently, which makes you feel tired and listless.

Post-viral fatigue
Some physical illnesses can cause extended periods of fatigue, such as glandular fever and ME (myalgic encephalomyelitis – also known as 'chronic fatigue syndrome').

Constipation

If your body's digestive system doesn't work efficiently – so you get constipated – you will feel sluggish, moody and generally off-colour.

Stress and depression

Stress and depression can also cause lethargy – and, conversely, being totally unmotivated and sloth-like will make you feel tired and depressed.

A BALANCED DIET

All of the above conditions can be improved through changes to your diet. If you often skip meals, don't eat regularly or go on fad diets, your energy levels will be reduced. A good, balanced diet is extremely important. If you think about it, your body needs fuel for energy. But not all fuel is the right fuel for optimum output and no fuel at all will result in you eventually grinding to a halt!

Later in this book, I shall give you details of menus and individual recipes that will help you to change your diet to build up and maintain your reserves of energy. But for now, it is sufficient to mention a few simple principles that you should remember when planning what to eat.

Cut down sugar and fat

It's not always what you don't eat that can cause the tiredness but what you eat too much of. For instance, a diet high in simple carbohydrates – that is, sugars – and fats will fill you up but make you feel bloated, sluggish and extremely fatigued after a quick energy boost. So if you are eating too many sugary cakes and biscuits (cookies), fatty snacks like crisps (chips) or pork pies or loads of chocolate bars, don't kid yourself that they will buck you up. They will give you a quick temporary lift but this will be followed by a major dip in energy levels.

Cut down caffeine

Contrary to what many people believe, caffeine doesn't always have the desired effect of waking you up. If you drink it in large quantities it will do exactly the opposite. One cup of black coffee will give you an instant lift, but six or more cups a day will make you tired and listless.

Eat a healthy, balanced diet

Whatever your problem, eating a healthy balanced diet with plenty of slow-release energy foods, fresh fruit and vegetables and cutting down on unnecessary fats, sugars and processed foods can make sure your energy intake is at its optimum so that you will feel better, healthier and more energetic. Cooking does destroy some of the vitamin and mineral content but by using a delicious blend of raw and quickly-cooked foods, my recipes will ensure that your body is provided with an excellent supply. The following chapters will give you some important food facts to help you maximise the benefits of the food you eat and fight that dreaded fatigue.

YOUR FATIGUE-FIGHTING DIET

Energy from your food is transported around your body as blood sugar. Some foods boost your blood-sugar levels quickly, but the levels then fall equally quickly. That will give you a boost of energy but leave you feeling worse than before. Other foods may take longer to get into your blood stream, but they stay there longer, too, so they are much more beneficial in helping to keep your blood sugar levels on an even keel, which is the aim if you are to stay alert and energetic. So the trick is to learn which groups of food have which effects, and stick to the good guys.

CHOOSING THE RIGHT FOOD

For the purposes of this book, I have divided foods into five main dietary groups.

Complex carbohydrates
These are found in starchy foods like bread, potatoes, pasta, rice, grains and wholegrain breakfast cereals. These give you fuel for energy, fill you up and keep you warm. They release energy slowly over a period of time, so will keep your body fuelled for longer.

Simple carbohydrates
These sugars are found in a natural form in some foods – such as fructose in fruit – but also in a refined form in all kinds of sweetened foods. Put bluntly, refined, added sugars are completely unnecessary. They give you a quick rush of blood sugar followed by a major 'dip', and that's not good news for fatigue fighters. Of course, you can have them as an occasional treat but you should not include them in your everyday regime.

Fruit and vegetables
These are good for you. You should aim to have five portions of fruit and vegetables a day to ensure you get all the fibre, vitamins and minerals you need to keep you healthy and alert.

Proteins
These are found in meat, pulses, seafood and eggs. They are vital for growth and repair of the body.

Fats
Your body needs some fat to keep the body and nervous system healthy. 'Essential fats', as they are known, are contained in oily fish, nuts, seeds and olive oil. However, whilst these are 'essential', your body does not need a great deal, so keep your intake within reasonable limits.

What the body does not need is extra fat, especially saturated fats (these are found in animal fats, and hard fats such as butter). Choose lean meat, don't eat the skin on poultry and put only a scraping of butter or other spread on bread.

START THE DAY RIGHT

If you wish to avoid fatigue, it is important that you give yourself the best possible start to your day. Breakfast literally means 'breaking your fast'. You may not have eaten anything since your evening meal and your body has then gone without food all through the night, which could be 12 hours or more. Although when sleeping you aren't using up huge amounts of energy, your body is burning calories – even if it's just to make you snore!

To keep your body fit and healthy, you must not miss breakfast. Most people who don't eat breakfast begin to feel tired by mid-morning and from then on they won't be functioning to their full potential even if they don't realise it.

However, it's no good just eating the first thing that comes to hand: the type of breakfast is important too. As I said in the introduction, a greasy fry-up won't keep you going after the initial boost, and a chocolate bar and a packet of crisps washed down with a coffee won't be any better. You need a meal high in complex carbohydrates for slow-release energy, combined with a little protein to help your body grow and repair itself and some fruits or vegetables for vital vitamins and minerals, to maintain your blood-sugar levels and keep you alert and functioning perfectly throughout the morning. If that sounds complicated, don't worry – it's not: a bowl of wholegrain cereal with a splash of milk and a glass of pure orange juice will do all of that!

EAT REGULAR AND SENSIBLE MEALS

It is important to keep your blood sugar at a steady level and to do this, you should eat sensible, regular meals. The timing is important too: your blood-sugar levels will begin to drop three or four hours after eating, and you will immediately start to feel tired. Small, frequent meals, which will provide you with a regular supply of energy throughout the day, are much better than starving all day and eating a single big meal in the evening.

Have a glass of pure fruit juice at breakfast, especially if you are having a fortified (preferably wholegrain) breakfast cereal. The vitamin C in the juice will help your body to absorb the iron in the cereal, ensuring you get the best out of both foods.

Don't skip lunch. Do make it a light, low-fat meal. High fat and sugar will mean a sleepy, sluggish afternoon!

Half of every meal should be made up of starchy foods, like bread, rice, pasta or potatoes. These will ensure a slow release of energy throughout the day. For best effects, try to use whole grains, wholewheat pasta and brown rice. These are not to everyone's taste, so you may prefer to use a combination of both. For example, brown basmati rice is great as an accompaniment, but doesn't make as good a risotto as the lovely polished Italian grains, so I use a mixture of brown and white grains in my diet. Both will give you slow-release energy; the brown grains give you more fibre as well.

Eat snacks that will boost your energy, not sap it. Avoid high-sugar biscuits (cookies), cakes and sweets (candies). Choose fresh or dried fruit, vegetables, nuts, seeds, wholegrain crackers and yoghurt. If you fancy something substantial, go for a currant bun rather than a Danish pastry, or a cheese scone (biscuit) instead of a chocolate brownie.

Don't eat big meals late at night. Your body won't be able to process the food properly or use the energy it could provide so you won't sleep well and you'll be tired the next day.

DOS AND DON'TS

There are two fatigue-fighting rules that I can't stress often enough. I've mentioned them once, but here they are again.

Cut the fat

Keep added fats to a minimum. All the fat your body requires can be found naturally in foods – everything from meat to dairy products, nuts and seeds – so you don't need to add more. A little monounsaturated oil, like olive, or polyunsaturated oil, like sunflower, is good for you but don't overdo it! Use low-fat sunflower, soya or olive oil spread instead of butter, and use it sparingly – just a scraping on bread and don't add it to vegetables after cooking.

For a serious reduction in your fat intake, eat only low-fat dairy products (cheese, creams, etc.); cut the fat off meat and don't eat the skin on poultry. Of course, you can still have the occasional treat. If, like me, you can't resist crackling with roast pork, you can still have a tiny bit once in a while!

Cut the sugar

Don't add sugar to your food or drinks. If you have to sweeten foods, use honey instead. It helps boost the supply of antioxidants in your body. This helps protect against the effects of free radicals, which prevent the body from getting the best out of food. Also, as honey is sweeter than sugar, you don't need so much of it.

When you need a sugar substitute – perhaps in a drink or, occasionally, in cooking – you can use artificial sweetener granules. These can be used spoon for spoon like sugar as the volume is similar, but they are much lighter, so don't try to use them by weight! Generally, however, I avoid them, as I am wary of what they contain.

THE WIDE-AWAKE NUTRIENTS

This quick-reference list contains all the good foods to fight fatigue. Aim to eat plenty of the following:

- **Stamina-building starches (complex carbohydrates)**
  Bread, pasta, rice, couscous, whole grains, potatoes

- **Anaemia-beating, iron- and folate-rich foods**
  Offal, dark green vegetables, beetroot, eggs, pulses, fortified breakfast cereals and bread, lean red meat (for iron), oily fish (iron) and wheatgerm (folate)

Note that **vitamin B12** (see below) is also vital in preventing anaemia.

- **Energy-releasing phosphorus**
  Found in lean meat and poultry, fish and shellfish, dairy products, nuts, seeds and whole grains

- **Energy-metabolising zinc**
  High levels in shellfish (particularly oysters!), red meat, peanuts and sunflower seeds

- **Vitality-inducing vitamin C**
  From fruit, particularly citrus, strawberries, black-currants, kiwis, guavas and (bell) peppers; also found in potatoes and green vegetables. Helps the body absorb iron too.

- **Energy-converting and -producing B-vitamin complex**
  Found in lean meat (particularly pork), offal, poultry, fish, nuts, seeds, pulses (dried peas, beans and lentils), eggs, dried fruit and fortified foods such as yeast extract and breakfast cereals

- **Drowsiness-fighting vitamin A**
  Found in eggs, dairy products, liver, oily fish and dark green, yellow and orange vegetables

- **Constipation-conquering fibre**
  Found in green, leafy vegetables, dried fruits, nuts, seeds, whole grains and the edible skin on fruit and vegetables

- **Wake-up water**
  The forgotten nutrient. Drink at least eight glasses a day – and that doesn't include what you have in tea or coffee.

FATIGUE-INDUCING FOODS

Many foods can actually make you feel more tired. Reduce the quantities of the following foods in your diet.

- **Energy-sapping added sugar (simple carbohydrates)**
  Found in cakes, biscuits (cookies), desserts, sugar-sweetened soft drinks, sweets (candies) and chocolate. It gives you a blast of instant energy but then leaves you feeling tired. The natural sugar in fruit, milk, etc. is okay as part of your daily food intake.

- **False-fix caffeine**
  Found in coffee, tea and colas. One cup can give you a quick buzz, six or more will leave you feeling exhausted. It also impairs sleep, leaving you feeling tired rather than refreshed the next day.

- **Sleep-inducing alcohol**
  One glass might act as a pick-you-up, but drink to excess and you'll feel worse than ever. Alcohol may send you off to sleep but it disturbs your sleep patterns, and will prevent your body from getting proper rest. Using it in cooking occasionally is okay because when boiled the alcohol content is removed.

EXERCISE – THE ENERGISER

Another way to help to beat fatigue is to take plenty of exercise. That may sound odd but it's true. It doesn't mean one extra-hard session a week at the gym but taking regular exercise – like walking briskly, playing sport or even gardening – that will stimulate your immune system and increase the amount of oxygen in your blood, leaving you feeling refreshed, not exhausted. If you incorporate a little more activity into your daily routine, you'll quickly feel the benefits.

YOUR SEVEN-DAY EATING PLAN

The previous chapters have covered some of the dietary rules you need to follow in order to fight fatigue. This one offers seven days of suggested menus that provide a simple guide to incorporating the rules into your daily diet. It will help you to get used to eating regularly, so it includes snacks as well as main meals, and shows you how fabulously well you can eat whilst remaining on the diet. You can, of course, mix and match any breakfast with any lunch and dinner recipes in the book.

For the most part, the plan uses my recipe suggestions but, obviously, you can use some of my healthy fast-food ideas too – such as Shredded Wheat for breakfast or a low-fat sandwich, bought ready-wrapped, for lunch. You don't have to eat the puddings – a piece of fresh fruit is by far the best option most of the time – but when you do want one, my recipes are guaranteed to make you feel good.

DAY 1

Breakfast	A glass of pure tomato juice
	High-energy Blueberry Orange and Sunflower Seed Muffin (see page 29)
	Coffee or tea
Mid-morning	A banana
Lunch	Mushroom and Leek Quiche (see page 54)
	Salad
	A satsuma
Mid-afternoon	Small slice of Carrot and Pecan Cake with Apple Cheese Frosting (see page 190)
Dinner	Steamed Trout with Asparagus on Chive Mash (see page 135)
	Baked Peach and Almond Brûlée (see page 173)

DAY 2

Breakfast   A glass of pure orange juice
Poached Eggs in Giant Mushrooms with
    Fresh Herbs (see page 21)
Tea or coffee

Mid-morning   An apple

Lunch   Tuna and Haricot Open Sandwich
    (see page 59)
A banana

Mid-afternoon Energy Boost Bar (see page 193)

Dinner   Turkey, Pineapple and Pepper Paella
    (see page 106)
Almond Jelly with Raspberry Coulis
    (see page 180)

DAY 3

Breakfast   A glass of pure apple juice
Oat and Apricot Porridge (see page 27)
Tea or coffee

Mid-morning   A plain digestive biscuit (graham cracker)

Lunch   Chinese Chicken Wrap (see page 62)
A nectarine

Mid-afternoon Date and Pistachio Square (see page 194)

Dinner   Grilled Mackerel with Mustard Seed and
    Raisin Couscous (see page 116)
Chilled Light Lemon Cheesecake
    (see page 178)

DAY 4

Breakfast	A glass of pure orange juice Crunchy Toasted Oat and Hazelnut Cereal (see page 28) with milk Tea or coffee
Mid-morning	Wholegrain crispbread with a scraping of Marmite
Lunch	French Onion Soup with Gruyère Croûtes (see page 38) Low-fat, sugar-free strawberry yoghurt with a handful of fresh strawberries
Mid-afternoon	Granary and Sesame Seed Bread Stick (see page 185)
Dinner	Seekh Kebabs with Fresh Mango Salsa (see page 82) and Tabbouleh (see page 154) Fruit and Nut Baked Apple (see page 168)

DAY 5

Breakfast	A glass of pure grapefruit juice Old English Kedgeree (see page 25) Tea or coffee
Mid-morning	An apple
Lunch	Cold Chilli Bean and Tuna Roll (see page 64) Low-fat sugar-free fromage frais
Mid-afternoon	Fruit and Fibre Scone (see page 184)
Dinner	Warm Sesame Chicken Salad (see page 100) Cinnamon Poached Pear (see page 172)

DAY 6

Breakfast	A slice of melon Scrambled Eggs with Soft Cheese and Tomatoes (see page 24) Tea or coffee
Mid-morning	A pear

Lunch	Prawn and Artichoke Mega Sandwich
	    (see page 63)
	Greek-style plain low-fat yoghurt with a
	    handful of raisins

Mid-afternoon	Peanut Sweetmeal Snack (see page 192)

Dinner	Grilled Oysters with Crème Fraîche
	    (see page 51)
	Steak Strips and Spinach Sizzle with
	    Crunchy Almond Ribbons (see page 72)
	Tropical Fruit Salad (see page 176)

DAY 7

Breakfast	A glass of pure pineapple juice Mega Muesli (see page 26) Tea or coffee
Mid-morning	A handful of raw peanuts
Lunch	Cheese Blusher (see page 65) An apple
Mid-afternoon	Mixed Fruit Flapjack (see page 189)

Dinner	Red-cooked Lamb with Green Thai Rice
	    (see page 84)
	Winter Fruit Compôte with Lime Cheese
	    (see page 175)

BASIC FOOD HYGIENE

A hygienic cook is a healthy cook – so please bear the following in mind when you're preparing food.

- Always wash your hands before starting.

- Always wash and dry fresh produce before use.

- Don't lick your fingers.

- Don't keep tasting and stirring with the same spoon. Use a clean spoon every time you taste the food.

- Never use a cloth to wipe down a chopping board you have been using for cutting up meat, for instance, then use the same one to wipe down your work surfaces – you will simply spread germs. Always wash your cloth well in hot, soapy water and, ideally, use an anti-bacterial kitchen cleaner on all surfaces too.

- Always transfer leftovers to a clean container and cover with a lid, clingfilm (plastic wrap) or foil. Leave until completely cold, then store in the fridge as soon as possible. Never put any warm food in the fridge.

- Don't put raw and cooked meat on the same shelf in the fridge. Store raw meat on the bottom shelf, so it can't drip over other foods. Keep all perishable foods wrapped separately. Don't overfill the fridge or it will remain too warm.

- When reheating food, always make sure it is piping hot throughout, never just lukewarm. To test made-up dishes, such as lasagne or a pie, insert a knife down through the centre. Leave for 5 seconds and remove. The blade should feel extremely hot. If not, heat a little longer.

- Don't re-freeze raw foods that have defrosted unless you cook them first. Never reheat previously cooked food more than once.

NOTES ON THE RECIPES

- All ingredients are given in imperial, metric and American measures. Follow one set only in a recipe. American terms are given in brackets.
- The ingredients are listed in the order in which they are used in the recipe.
- All spoon measures are level: 1 tsp=5 ml; 1 tbsp=15 ml
- Eggs are medium unless otherwise stated.
- Always wash, peel, core and seed, if necessary, fresh produce before use.
- Seasoning and the use of strongly flavoured ingredients such as garlic or chillies are very much a matter of personal taste. Taste the food as you cook and adjust to suite your own palate.
- Fresh herbs are great for garnishing and adding flavour. Pots of them are available in all good supermarkets. Keep your favourite ones on the windowsill and water regularly. Jars of ready-prepared herbs, like coriander (cilantro) and lemon grass, and frozen ones – chopped parsley in particular – are also very useful. If you substitute dried for fresh, use only about one-third – or less – as dried herbs are very pungent.
- All can and packet sizes are approximate as they vary from brand to brand. For example, if I call for a 400 g/14 oz/large can of tomatoes and yours is a 397 g can, that's fine.
- Cooking times are approximate and should be used as a guide only. Always check food is piping hot and cooked through before serving.
- Always preheat the oven and cook on the shelf just above the centre unless otherwise stated (note that fan ovens do not need preheating and the positioning is not so crucial).
- Instead of butter or ordinary margarine, use a low-fat sunflower, soya or olive oil spread suitable for cooking and spreading.
- Use skimmed or semi-skimmed milk (**not** full-cream) and choose low-fat varieties of cheese, cream and yoghurt, when appropriate.

BOOSTING BREAKFASTS

Breakfast is a very important meal if
you want to feel fit, healthy and wide
awake. Always have a glass of pure fruit
juice unless your breakfast includes
fresh fruit. If you like to have tea or
coffee, make it caffeine-free and whiten
with skimmed (preferably) or semi-
skimmed milk.

Poached Eggs in Giant Mushrooms with Fresh Herbs

Mushrooms are a good source of phosphorus, B-vitamins and folate. Baked and served with iron-rich eggs on a delicious slice of granary toast, they make the perfect start to the day and take very little time to prepare. NB: Do make sure the mushrooms are not too open, or the eggs will slide off!

SERVES 4

---

4 very large open-cup mushrooms

A small pinch of celery salt

15 ml/1 tbsp chopped fresh thyme

90 ml/6 tbsp water

4 eggs

4 slices of granary bread

A scraping of low-fat sunflower, soya or olive oil spread

15 ml/1 tbsp chopped fresh parsley

---

1 Peel the mushrooms and remove any stalks. Sprinkle with a very little celery salt and the thyme.

2 Put the water in a large non-stick frying pan (skillet) and lay the mushrooms, gill-sides up, in the pan. Bring to the boil.

3 Break an egg into a cup and slide into one of the mushrooms. Repeat with the remaining eggs and mushrooms.

4 Cover the pan with a lid or foil, turn down the heat to moderate and poach for 4–5 minutes until the mushrooms are cooked and the eggs are just set. Cook a little longer if you like your eggs hard.

5 Meanwhile, toast the bread and add a scraping of spread. Place on warm plates. Lift the mushrooms out of the pan with a fish slice and place on the toast. Sprinkle with the parsley and serve.

Potato and Bacon Omelette Wedges

If you have an automatic oven, you can prepare the dish the night before, then put it in a lightly greased baking dish and place it in the oven, set to bake at 190°C/375°F/gas 5/fan oven 170°C for about 35 minutes. You can used drained canned potatoes, if you prefer. A 275 g/10 oz/medium can is just the right quantity.

SERVES 4

15 g/½ oz/1 tbsp low-fat sunflower, soya or olive oil spread

2 rashers (slices) of extra-lean smoked back bacon, finely diced

1 small onion, sliced

2 cooked potatoes, sliced

6 eggs

90 ml/6 tbsp water

A pinch of salt

Freshly ground black pepper

To serve:

Sliced tomatoes

1 Heat the low-fat spread in a medium-sized non-stick frying pan (skillet). Add the bacon and onion and cook, stirring, until the bacon and onion are golden.

2 Add the sliced potatoes and mix gently.

3 Beat the eggs and water together with the salt and lots of pepper. Pour into the pan. Cook, lifting the edges from time to time to allow the uncooked egg to run underneath, until the egg is almost set.

4 Preheat the grill (broiler). Place the pan under the grill to brown the surface.

5 Serve cut into wedges with sliced tomatoes.

Eggs Florentine on Granary

Spinach is an excellent source of iron and folate (amongst other things) and eggs are rich in vitamin A. Bathed in a smooth cheese sauce on good wholegrain bread, they will help to keep you wide awake and sustained all morning.

SERVES 4

450 g/1 lb spinach

150 ml/¹/₄ pt/²/₃ cup low-fat crème fraîche

A little freshly grated nutmeg

Salt and freshly ground black pepper

100 g/4 oz/¹/₂ cup low-fat cheese spread

60 ml/4 tbsp milk

4 eggs

15 ml/1 tbsp lemon juice or white wine vinegar

4 slices of granary bread

---

1 Wash the spinach. Place in a covered pan with no extra water and cook for 5 minutes. Drain thoroughly in a colander and snip with scissors to chop. Return to the pan and stir in 60 ml/4 tbsp of the crème fraîche, a little nutmeg, salt and pepper. Reheat.

2 Meanwhile, put the cheese spread, the remaining crème fraîche and the milk into a saucepan. Heat gently, stirring with a wire whisk, until melted but do not allow to boil.

3 Poach the eggs in an egg poacher or in a pan of gently simmering water with the lemon juice or vinegar added for 3–4 minutes until cooked to your liking.

4 Toast the bread. Place on small warm plates and top with the creamed spinach. Top each with a poached egg. Preheat the grill (broiler).

5 Spoon the cheese sauce over the eggs. Place under the grill for about 2 minutes to brown the top. Serve immediately.

Scrambled Eggs
with Soft Cheese and Tomatoes

This is based on a recipe from the Victorian era – when they really knew how to enjoy breakfast. The cheese and mustard enrich the eggs and add extra wake-up nutrients. The rich, creamy concoction is served on a bed of tomatoes on lightly toasted wholemeal bread – the perfect start to a busy day.

SERVES 4

---

4 slices of wholemeal bread

4 tomatoes, sliced

A small knob of low-fat sunflower, soya or olive oil spread

6 eggs

45 ml/3 tbsp milk

10 ml/2 tsp made English mustard

100 g/4 oz/½ cup low-fat soft cheese

A pinch of salt

Freshly ground black pepper

1 Preheat the grill (broiler) and toast the bread on one side. Turn over and lay the tomatoes on top. Grill (broil) until the tomatoes have softened, then turn off the grill. Leave the toasts under the warm grill, so that they do not become cold.

2 Meanwhile, melt the low-fat spread in a non-stick saucepan. Beat together the eggs, milk, mustard and cheese, season with a pinch of salt and lots of pepper and pour into the pan. Cook over a gentle heat, stirring all the time, until the eggs are just set but still creamy. Do not allow to boil.

3 Transfer the tomato toasts to warm plates. Spoon the eggs on top and serve straight away.

Old English Kedgeree

This makes a delicious lunch or supper but is also the perfect combination of protein and carbohydrates to set you up for a busy morning. You can make it the night before, then reheat it either in the microwave or in a saucepan, with a couple of tablespoons of milk to keep it moist.

SERVES 4

3 eggs, scrubbed under cold water

225 g/8 oz/1 cup long-grain rice

Salt

5 ml/1 tsp ground turmeric

225 g/8 oz smoked haddock fillet, skinned

100 g/4 oz/1 cup frozen peas

2.5 ml/¹/₂ tsp ground cumin

45 ml/3 tbsp chopped fresh parsley

Freshly ground black pepper

1 Put the eggs in a large saucepan of water. Bring to the boil.

2 Add the rice, a pinch of salt and the turmeric. Stir, then cook over a high heat for 5 minutes. Add the fish and peas and cook for a further 5 minutes or until the rice and fish are tender.

3 Lift out the eggs and fish. Put the eggs in a bowl of cold water. Drain the rice and peas in a colander and return to the pan. Stir in the cumin.

4 Remove the skin from the fish and break the flesh into chunks. Add to the rice.

5 Shell the eggs and cut into chunks. Add to the rice.

6 Add the parsley and lots of pepper. Stir gently over a fairly low heat until piping hot.

7 Pile on to warm plates and serve.

Mega Muesli

There are plenty of different mueslis available in the shops now but this one not only has the perfect balance of fruits, nuts and seeds, but also, spoon for spoon, is much cheaper. Try not to add sugar – it doesn't need it – but if you must have it slightly sweeter, drizzle your portion with 5 ml/1 tsp honey.

MAKES ABOUT 1 KG/2¼ LB

350 g/12 oz/3 cups rolled oats

100 g/4 oz/1 cup wheat bran

100 g/4 oz/1 cup brown rice flakes

100 g/4 oz/²/₃ cup raisins or sultanas (golden raisins)

100 g/4 oz/²/₃ cup dried banana slices

100 g/4 oz/1 cup sunflower seeds

100 g/4 oz/1 cup toasted chopped mixed nuts

10 ml/2 tsp mixed (apple-pie) spice

To serve:

Milk or plain low-fat yoghurt

1 Mix all the ingredients together and store in an airtight container.

2 Serve with milk or yoghurt.

Oat and Apricot Porridge

Oats are good for lowering cholesterol as well as being a good source of sustainable energy. Blended with dried apricots for added nutrients, this makes a substantial health-giving breakfast. It is also easy to make in the microwave: use a large bowl so it doesn't boil over during cooking and cook for 5–10 minutes, stirring from time to time.

SERVES 4

---

175 g/6 oz/1½ cups quick-cook rolled oats

1 litre/1¾ pts/4¼ cups milk and water, mixed

A pinch of salt

175 g/6 oz/1 cup chopped ready-to-eat dried apricots

To serve:

Milk or low-fat crème fraîche

---

1 Blend the oats with the milk and water in a non-stick saucepan. Bring to the boil, stirring.

2 Stir in the apricots, then turn down the heat and simmer for 5–10 minutes until thick and creamy, stirring frequently.

3 Spoon into bowls and serve with milk or crème fraîche.

Crunchy Toasted Oat and Hazelnut Cereal

This is as good as any bought crunchy cereal but as it contains no added sugar and only a fairly small amount of honey, it is an even better source of slow-release energy. Try serving it topped with low-fat yoghurt or buttermilk for a change from skimmed or semi-skimmed milk.

MAKES ABOUT 700 G/1½ LB

225 g/8 oz/2 cups rolled oats

100 g/4 oz/1 cup buckwheat grains

100 g/4 oz/1 cup chopped hazelnuts (filberts)

100 g/4 oz/1 cup pumpkin seeds

100 g /4 oz/1 cup sesame seeds

90 ml/6 tbsp clear honey

60 ml/4 tbsp water

50 g/2 oz/¼ cup low-fat sunflower, soya or olive oil spread, melted

To serve:

Milk

---

1 Preheat the oven to 160°C/325°F/gas 3/fan oven 145°C. Mix the dry ingredients together.

2 Blend the honey with the water and melted spread and mix in thoroughly. Spread the mixture out on a baking (cookie) sheet.

3 Bake in the oven for about 1 hour until golden and crisp. Leave to cool.

4 Crumble into an airtight container.

5 Serve with milk.

High-energy Blueberry Orange and Sunflower Seed Muffins

These wholemeal muffins, full of fruits and seeds, make an ideal start to the day – or a perfect tea-time treat. If you don't have large muffin tins, make smaller ones in tartlet tins, lined with paper cake cases, and cook for only 20 minutes.

MAKES 12

Finely grated zest and juice of 1 large orange

Boiling water

100 g/4 oz/²/₃ cup dried blueberries

40 g/1¹/₂ oz/3 tbsp low-fat sunflower, soya or olive oil spread

50 g/2 oz/¹/₂ cup sunflower seeds

75 g/3 oz/¹/₃ cup thick honey

225 g/8 oz/2 cups self-raising (self-rising) wholemeal flour

5 ml/1 tsp baking powder

1 egg, beaten

1 Preheat the oven to 180°C/350°F/gas 4/fan oven 160°C. Put the orange zest and juice in a measuring jug and make up to 300 ml/¹/₂ pt/1¹/₄ cups with boiling water.

2 Add the blueberries and the spread. Leave to soak until the liquid is just warm.

3 Tip the mixture into a bowl and add all the remaining ingredients. Mix together thoroughly.

4 Lightly grease non-stick muffin tins (pans). Spoon the mixture into the tins (they should be nearly full). Bake in the oven for about 25–30 minutes or until they are risen and the centres spring back when lightly pressed. Transfer to a wire rack to cool.

5 Serve warm or cold.

Sweet Spiced Oat and Parsnip Muffins

These gorgeous, highly nutritious bakes will keep you alert for hours! You can ring the changes, using carrots instead of parsnips and wheat bran instead of oat, and experiment with ground cinnamon instead of mace.

MAKES 12

---

1 large parsnip, grated

75 g/3 oz/⅓ cup thick honey

100 g/4 oz/1 cup self-raising (self-rising) wholemeal flour

100 g/4 oz/1 cup oat bran

15 ml/1 tbsp baking powder

75 g/3 oz/¾ cup chopped walnuts

75 g/3 oz/½ cup sultanas (golden raisins)

2.5 ml/½ tsp ground mace

60 ml/4 tbsp sunflower oil

150 ml/¼ pt/⅔ cup plain low-fat yoghurt

150 ml/¼ pt/⅔ cup milk

1 egg, beaten

---

1 Lightly grease the sections of non-stick muffin tins (pans). Preheat the oven to 180°C/350°F/gas 4/fan oven 160°C.

2 Mix all the ingredients together and beat well.

3 Spoon the mixture into the tins (they should be nearly full) and bake in the oven for 25–30 minutes until they are risen and the centres spring back when lightly pressed.

4 Cool slightly, then turn out on to a wire rack to cool completely. Serve warm or cold.

Quick-fix Breakfasts

This list provides some ideas for excellent, simple-to-make, super-quick starts to the day. As before, have a glass of pure fruit juice as well.

- 1 or 2 Shredded Wheat (or Weetabix), topped with a handful of tropical fruit and nut mix and milk

- 1 or 2 Weetabix, spread with a scraping of low-fat sunflower, soya or olive oil spread and honey or Marmite

- A bowl of bran flakes with a sliced banana, topped with a little milk and a spoonful of Greek-style low-fat yoghurt

- Oat porridge, served with buttermilk and a small teaspoon of honey

- A bagel, split, toasted, spread with low-fat soft cheese and topped with a few crushed strawberries, raspberries or blueberries. If more convenient, use fruit canned in natural juice (drain it well) or thawed frozen fruit

- An English muffin (preferably wholemeal), split, toasted and filled with a slice of Edam cheese and a poached egg

- Half a grapefruit, topped with a small teaspoon of clear honey and grilled (broiled) until turning golden, followed by one or two slices of wholemeal or granary toast and a scraping of peanut butter

- A boiled or poached egg, wholemeal toast with a scraping of low-fat sunflower, soya or olive oil spread and a scraping of Marmite

- 1 or 2 eggs, scrambled with a dash of milk and a small knob of low-fat sunflower, soya or olive oil spread, on granary toast

- Hot, unsweetened, instant oat cereal, with a handful of raisins or a trickle of clear honey or a spoonful of pure pear and apple spread

BREAKFAST SMOOTHIES

If you really can't face sitting down to a meal when you've just got up, or never have enough time for breakfast, a smoothie is just the thing for you to start the day. They are ultra-simple to make – just whizz one up in a blender – and take no time to drink. And they'll keep your concentration levels up for several hours! My son makes them often, but doubles the quantity – mind you, he is 1.93 m/6 ft 4 in tall!

Banana Bonanza

This is the perfect morning drink – thick, fruity and filling. If your banana is still a little green, add 5 ml/1 tsp clear honey. Try adding a low-fat fruit yoghurt instead of half the milk to ring the changes too.

SERVES 1

1 large ripe banana

175 ml /6 fl oz/³/₄ cup cold milk

15 ml/1 tbsp instant oat cereal

1 Peel and break the banana into pieces.
2 Put into a blender with the milk and oat cereal and blend until thick, frothy and smooth.
3 Pour into a large glass.

Tomato and Orange Tantaliser

Another zingy booster to get you ready to roll. Packed with vitamin C, plus the added goodness from the almonds, this is a winning wake-up drink. Add some crunchy breadsticks to sustain your energies even longer (see the recipe on page 185 or buy them ready-made, if you prefer).

SERVES 1

---

250 ml/8 fl oz/1 cup tomato juice

150 ml/¼ pt/⅔ cup pure orange juice

30 ml/2 tbsp ground almonds

Finely grated zest and juice of ½ lime or ½ small lemon

To serve:

Granary bread sticks

---

1 Put all the ingredients in a blender and blend until smooth.

2 Pour into a large glass and serve with bread sticks.

Mango and Kiwi Smoothie

This is a very refreshing start to the morning! The fruits give you a good blast of vitamins and minerals, including phosphorus and vitamin C. Try using a papaya or a couple of nectarines instead of the mango for a change.

SERVES 1

---

1 small or ½ large ripe mango

1 ripe kiwi fruit

150 ml/¼ pt/⅔ cup thick plain low-fat yoghurt

150 ml/¼ pt/⅔ cup pure apple juice

15 ml/1 tbsp wheatgerm

---

1 Peel the mango and cut all the flesh off the stone (pit). Place in the blender.

2 Peel the kiwi fruit and add.

3 Add all the remaining ingredients and blend until smooth.

4 Pour into a large glass.

Avocado Awakener

This is for those of you who prefer something savoury. It is a bit like guacamole in a glass, and it makes a perfect wake-up drink. Avocados are high in protein and a great source of vitamins and minerals, particularly phosphorus. They are also rich in monounsaturated fat – which won't raise your cholesterol levels at all.

SERVES 1
1 slice of bread
150 ml/¹/₄ pt/²/₃ cup water
150 ml/¹/₄ pt/²/₃ cup passata (sieved tomatoes)
1 small avocado (or ¹/₂ large), peeled and stoned (pitted)
1 spring onion (scallion), trimmed and chopped
A dash of Worcestershire sauce
A pinch of salt
A pinch of cayenne or chilli powder
Freshly ground black pepper
Ice cubes (optional)

1 Break up the bread, place in a blender, add the water and soak for a minute or two.

2 Add the remaining ingredients and blend until smooth. Taste and add more seasoning, if necessary.

3 Pour into a large glass. Add ice cubes, if liked.

SUSTAINING SOUPS

These soups are substantial enough to
be eaten on their own for lunch or
supper but could also be served before
a light main course, such as a salad.
They all have an excellent balance of
nutrients to keep you feeling sustained
but wide awake.

Parsnip, Lemon and Coriander Soup

Parsnips are a good source of numerous minerals and vitamins as well as being high in complex carbohydrates for sustained energy. Blended subtly with coriander and lemon, they make a smooth, mouth-watering soup, ideal to be served for lunch or supper.

SERVES 6

25 g/1 oz/2 tbsp low-fat sunflower, soya or olive oil spread

1 large onion, roughly chopped

2 parsnips, diced

1 large potato, diced

Finely grated zest and juice of 1 small lemon

1.5 litres/2½ pts/6 cups vegetable stock, made with 2 stock cubes

45 ml/3 tbsp fine oatmeal or unsweetened instant oat cereal

1 bay leaf

30 ml/2 tbsp chopped fresh coriander (cilantro)

30 ml/2 tbsp chopped fresh parsley

45 ml/3 tbsp dried milk powder (non-fat dried milk)

Salt and freshly ground black pepper

30 ml/6 tsp low-fat crème fraîche, for garnishing

To serve:

Granary rolls

1 Melt the low-fat spread in a large saucepan. Add the onion and fry (sauté), stirring, for 2 minutes until softened but not browned.

2 Stir the parsnips and potato into the pan and cook for 1 minute.

3 Add the lemon zest and juice, the stock, oatmeal and bay leaf. Stir well. Bring to the boil, reduce the heat, part-cover and simmer gently for 20 minutes or until everything is tender.

4 Liquidise in a blender or food processor with the herbs and milk powder, then return to the pan. Season to taste and reheat.

5 Ladle into warm bowls and top each with a teaspoon of crème fraîche.

6 Serve with granary rolls.

French Onion Soup
with Gruyère Croûtes

This classic soup is hard to beat. Onions are renowned for their health-giving properties and here they are cooked to golden richness, then simmered in stock to form a nourishing tasty soup, topped with bread and creamy Swiss cheese for long-term energy, to make a perfect meal.

SERVES 6

---

15 ml/1 tbsp olive oil

A knob of low-fat sunflower, soya or olive oil spread

450 g/1 lb onions, halved and thinly sliced

15 ml/1 tbsp clear honey

1.2 litres/2 pts/5 cups vegetable stock, made with 2 stock cubes

Salt and freshly ground black pepper

6 slices of French bread

100 g/4 oz/1 cup low-fat Gruyère cheese, finely grated

1 Heat the oil and the low-fat spread in a large saucepan. Add the onions and fry (sauté), stirring, over a moderate heat for 5 minutes until lightly golden.

2 Add the honey and continue to fry for a further 2–3 minutes until richly caramelised (take care not to burn it).

3 Add the stock, bring back to the boil, reduce the heat and simmer for 15 minutes. Season to taste.

4 Meanwhile, toast the bread on both sides. Pile the cheese on top, pressing on well.

5 Ladle the soup into warm, flameproof bowls. Float a piece of the cheese toast on top of each and place under a preheated grill (broiler) for about 3 minutes until the cheese melts and bubbles, and serve.

Chicken and Vegetable Broth with Barley

Another soup packed with vitamins and minerals, plus a good handful of barley for sustained energy – this is real comfort food at its best. If you have a food processor, you can chop the onion in it, then put on the grating attachment and prepare all the other vegetables.

SERVES 4

---

50 g/2 oz/¹⁄₂ cup pearl barley

1 onion, finely chopped

1 carrot, coarsely grated

1 potato, coarsely grated

1 turnip, coarsely grated

1 skinless chicken breast

900 ml/1¹⁄₂ pts/3 cups water

1 bouquet garni sachet

2 chicken stock cubes

Salt and freshly ground black pepper

30 ml/2 tbsp chopped fresh parsley

---

1 Put the pearl barley, onion, carrot, potato and turnip in a saucepan.

2 Add the chicken, water, bouquet garni sachet and stock cubes and season lightly.

3 Bring to the boil, then reduce the heat, part-cover and simmer for 30 minutes. Discard the bouquet garni.

4 Lift the chicken out, chop finely and return to the pan. Taste and re-season. Add the parsley.

5 Heat through and serve.

Mediterranean Vegetable Soup

Packed with many nutrients you need to keep you healthy and alert, this soup has a wonderful flavour and rich aroma. You can adjust the selection of vegetables, depending on what you have available.

SERVES 6

1 onion, finely chopped

1 garlic clove, crushed

15 ml/1 tbsp olive oil

1 green (bell) pepper, finely chopped

1 red pepper, finely chopped

1 large courgette (zucchini), finely chopped

1 small aubergine (eggplant), finely chopped

1 × 400 g/14 oz/large can of chopped tomatoes

1 × 425 g/15 oz/large can of cannellini beans, drained

30 ml/2 tbsp tomato purée (paste)

1 litre/1³/₄ pts/4¹/₄ cups chicken or vegetable stock, made with 2 stock cubes

2.5 ml/¹/₂ tsp dried oregano

Salt and freshly ground black pepper

2 vermicelli nests, crushed

15 ml/1 tbsp chopped fresh basil

50 g/2 oz/¹/₂ cup freshly grated Parmesan cheese

1 In a large saucepan, fry (sauté) the onion and garlic in the oil for 2 minutes, stirring occasionally, until softened but not browned.

2 Add all the remaining ingredients except the basil and cheese. Bring to the boil, reduce the heat, part-cover and simmer gently for 20 minutes until the vegetables are tender. Taste and re-season, if necessary.

3 Ladle into warm, wide shallow soup bowls, sprinkle with the basil and cheese and serve hot.

Spinach and Broad Bean Soup with Yoghurt

Green, smooth and utterly delicious, this soup will keep you sustained for several hours. High in nutrients and flavour, it is perfect for lunch or supper. It is so simple to make, you can throw it together for a quick meal, but it is good enough to serve to guests, perhaps garnished with some fresh chopped herbs.

SERVES 4

1 large onion, chopped

1 large potato, finely chopped

225 g/8 oz frozen broad (fava) beans

225 g/8 oz frozen spinach

900 ml/1½ pts/3¾ cups vegetable or chicken stock, made with 2 stock cubes

Salt and freshly ground black pepper

Freshly grated nutmeg

60 ml/4 tbsp plain low-fat yoghurt

1   Put all the ingredients except the nutmeg and yoghurt in a saucepan. Bring to the boil over a high heat, then reduce the heat until gently bubbling around the edges, part-cover and cook for 10 minutes until everything is tender.

2   Purée the soup in a blender or food processor and return to the pan. Add salt, pepper and nutmeg to taste. Reheat.

3   Ladle into warm bowls and add a spoonful of yoghurt to each.

4   Serve hot.

Smoked Haddock and Potato Bisque with Poached Eggs

The eggs in this delicious soup provide plenty of fatigue-fighting iron and vitamin A. It's a rich and delicious soup that tastes great with a slice of wholemeal or granary bread. If you are looking for something slightly less substantial, however, you can serve it without the eggs.

SERVES 6

1 leek, finely chopped

15 g/½ oz/1 tbsp low-fat sunflower, soya or olive oil spread

1 large potato, finely diced

225 g/8 oz undyed smoked haddock

750 ml/1¼ pts/3 cups fish stock, made with 1 stock cube

150 ml/¼ pt/⅔ cups pure apple juice

1 bouquet garni sachet

Freshly ground black pepper

60 ml/4 tbsp dried milk powder (non-fat dry milk)

150 ml/¼ pt/⅔ cups water

25 ml/1½ tbsp cornflour (cornstarch)

6 eggs

15 ml/1 tbsp wine vinegar

30 ml/2 tbsp chopped fresh parsley, for garnishing

1 Place the leek in a large saucepan with the low-fat spread and fry (sauté), stirring, for 2 minutes, until softened but not browned.

2 Stir in the potato and cook gently for 30 seconds.

3 Add the fish, stock, apple juice and bouquet garni. Season lightly with pepper. Bring to the boil, reduce the heat, part-cover and simmer very gently for 20 minutes until the potato and fish are tender.

4 Carefully lift the fish out of the pan with a draining spoon. Remove the skin and any bones and discard. Flake the fish. Discard the bouquet garni.

5 Blend the milk powder and water with the cornflour until smooth. Stir into the pan. Bring to the boil and cook for 1 minute, stirring. Add the flaked fish.

6 Poach the eggs in gently simmering water to which the vinegar has been added, or in an egg poacher, for 3–5 minutes until cooked to your liking.

7 Ladle the soup into warm bowls and slide an egg into each bowl. Garnish with chopped parsley before serving.

Spiced Lentil and Tomato Soup

Lentils are a great source of protein and complex carbohydrates as well as minerals and vitamins, including iron, phosphorus, zinc and some B-vitamins. Blended with tomatoes, for a boost of vitamin C, and judiciously seasoned, they make a warming and delicious soup.

SERVES 4

---

10 ml/2 tsp olive oil

1 onion, chopped

1 carrot, chopped

5 ml/1 tsp ground cumin

100 g/4 oz/²⁄₃ cup red lentils

600 ml/1 pt/2½ cups chicken or vegetable stock, made with 1 stock cube

1 × 400 g/14 oz/large can of chopped tomatoes

30 ml/2 tbsp tomato purée (paste)

5 ml/1 tsp clear honey

Salt and freshly ground black pepper

15 ml/1 tbsp chopped fresh coriander (cilantro), for garnishing

---

1 Heat the oil in a saucepan over a moderate heat. Add the onion and carrot and fry (sauté), stirring, for 2 minutes, until softened but not browned. Stir in the cumin and cook for 1 minute.

2 Add all the remaining ingredients. Bring to the boil, reduce the heat, part-cover and simmer for about 30 minutes until the lentils are completely soft. Liquidise in a blender or food processor. Return to the pan and heat through.

3 Taste the soup and re-season, if necessary. Ladle into warm bowls and garnish each with a sprinkling of chopped coriander.

4 Serve hot.

Almond Chicken Soup with Rice

Almonds and chicken for protein, multi-vitamins and minerals, plus rice for sustained energy – this is a worthy fatigue-fighting combination. It makes a rich and tasty soup that is easy to prepare and will keep you going for hours.

SERVES 6

---

100 g/4 oz/1 cup ground almonds

1.2 litres/2 pts/5 cups hot chicken stock, made with 2 stock cubes

Salt and freshly ground white pepper

100 g/4 oz cooked chicken, finely chopped

50 g/2 oz/¼ cup long-grain rice

150 ml/¼ pt/⅔ cup low-fat crème fraîche

15 ml/1 tbsp chopped fresh parsley, for garnishing

---

1 Put the almonds in a saucepan. Add about 300 ml/ ½ pt/1¼ cups of the hot stock, whisking all the time, until the mixture is smooth. Whisk in the remaining stock and a little salt and pepper.

2 Bring to the boil over a high heat, reduce the heat until bubbling gently around the edges and cook for 10 minutes.

3 Add the chicken and rice and cook for a further 10 minutes. Stir in the crème fraîche and heat through but do not boil. Taste and re-season, if necessary.

4 Serve straight away, garnished with chopped parsley.

Green Pepper Borsch

Rich in iron, folate and vitamin C as well as loads of other nutrients, this deep red soup has bags of flavour too. You can enjoy it steaming hot on a cold winter's day or chilled and served with a few floating ice cubes in the height of summer. Either way, it's delicious.

SERVES 4

---

2 celery sticks, coarsely grated, discarding the strings

2 carrots, coarsely grated

1 small onion, grated

1 green (bell) pepper, grated

3 cooked beetroot (red beets), grated

900 ml/1½ pts/3¾ cups beef stock, made with 2 stock cubes

15 ml/1 tbsp red wine vinegar

Salt and freshly ground black pepper

60 ml/4 tbsp low-fat crème fraîche

1 Put the grated vegetables in a saucepan with the stock, vinegar and some salt and pepper.

2 Cook over a high heat until boiling.

3 Turn down the heat until gently bubbling around the edges, then part-cover the pan with a lid and cook gently for 20 minutes. Taste and re-season, if necessary.

4 Ladle into warm bowls and top each with a spoonful of crème fraîche before serving.

ENERGISING STARTERS AND LIGHT MEALS

Whether you want a quick lunch or supper dish, a snack to eat 'on the hoof' or a simple starter to tickle the taste buds, there's something to suit you in this chapter's selection. All the recipes include the ideal ingredients to keep you alert and focused.

Smoky Aubergine Dip with Little Gems

Aubergines have a little of almost everything in them, nutritionally speaking. They are also the perfect vehicle for other good things, such as garlic, tomatoes and olive oil. Served with wholemeal pittas, they make a perfectly balanced snack or starter with a delightful Mediterranean touch.

SERVES 4

1 large aubergine (eggplant)

1 spring onion (scallion), very finely chopped

1 small garlic clove, crushed

2 large ripe tomatoes, skinned, seeded and chopped

45 ml/3 tbsp olive oil

Lemon juice, to taste

Salt and freshly ground black pepper

15 ml/1 tbsp chopped fresh parsley

2 little gem lettuces

4 wholemeal pitta breads

1 Preheat the grill (broiler). Grill (broil) the aubergine for about 15 minutes, turning occasionally, until the skin blackens and the flesh feels soft when squeezed.

2 When cool enough to handle, peel off the skin and discard, then chop the flesh finely and place in a bowl.

3 Mix in the spring onion, garlic and tomatoes.

4 Add the oil, a drop or two at a time, stirring briskly with a wooden spoon after each addition until the mixture is glistening but still quite thick. Add lemon juice, salt and pepper to taste. Spoon into four small pots and chill.

5 Pull the lettuces into separate leaves, wash and dry well. Arrange the leaves on plates with a pot of dip in the middle.

6 Warm the pitta breads and cut into fingers. Put the bread fingers to one side of each plate.

7 Serve while still warm.

Tomato, Egg and Mozzarella Platter

All the ingredients of this simple but delicious platter will keep you alert and vibrant. The combination of flavours, colours and textures is a delight to look at – and to eat.

SERVES 4
60 ml/4 tbsp pine nuts
2 × 125 g/4½ oz low-fat Mozzarella cheeses
4 hard-boiled (hard-cooked) eggs, shelled and sliced
8 tomatoes, sliced
12 stoned (pitted) black olives
8 large basil leaves, torn
30 ml/2 tbsp olive oil
15 ml/1 tbsp balsamic vinegar
Freshly ground black pepper
To serve:
Warm ciabatta bread

1 Heat a frying pan (skillet). Add the pine nuts and toss until golden. Tip out of the pan immediately so they don't burn.

2 Slice each Mozzarella cheese into six slices. Arrange with the slices of egg and tomato, overlapping each other attractively, on four serving plates. Scatter the pine nuts, olives and basil over.

3 Trickle the oil and vinegar over the salads and sprinkle with pepper.

4 Serve with ciabatta bread.

Warm Chicken Livers with Blueberries

Iron-rich chicken livers blended with vitamin-packed blueberries and folate-rich salad leaves make a tasty, nutritious and stimulating starter or light lunch.

SERVES 4

---

200 g/7 oz chicken livers

15 g/½ oz/1 tbsp low-fat sunflower, soya or olive oil spread

Salt and freshly ground black pepper

100 g/4 oz blueberries

15 ml/1 tbsp pure apple juice

100 g/4 oz mixed salad leaves

15 ml/1 tbsp balsamic vinegar

45 ml /3 tbsp olive oil

5 ml/1 tsp grainy mustard

To serve:

Small wholemeal rolls

---

1 Trim the chicken livers. Heat the spread in a non-stick frying pan (skillet) over a fairly high heat. Add the chicken livers and a little seasoning and stir-fry for 4–5 minutes until just cooked but still soft.

2 Add the blueberries and apple juice to the pan juices, cover with a lid, turn down the heat to fairly low and cook gently for 1 minute.

3 Meanwhile, put the leaves in a bowl. In a small bowl, whisk together the vinegar, oil, mustard and some salt and pepper with a wire whisk. Add to the salad and toss with your hands or a spoon and fork to coat the leaves.

4 Pile on to plates. Top with the chicken livers, blueberries and their juices.

5 Serve warm with small wholemeal rolls.

Grilled Oysters
with Crème Fraîche

Oysters are one of the best sources of zinc as well as containing other vitamins and minerals. Grilled with low-fat crème fraîche, a little cheese and a dash of Tabasco sauce, they are truly in a league all of their own. Great for the brain and, apparently, for the libido too!

SERVES 4

16 fresh oysters in their shells

Freshly ground black pepper

Tabasco sauce

90 ml/6 tbsp low-fat crème fraîche

90 ml/6 tbsp freshly grated Parmesan cheese

To serve:

Oatcakes (see page 183 or buy ready-made)

1 Shuck (open) the oysters. To do this, hold each oyster firmly in one hand. Insert a sharp, pointed knife between the two shells, near the hinge. Pushing against the hinge, twist the knife until the hinge breaks.

2 Carefully open the oyster, taking care not to spill the juice, and loosen it from its shell.

3 Preheat the grill (broiler). Remove the grill rack and put the oysters in their half shells in the grill pan. Add a good grinding of pepper and a dash of Tabasco sauce.

3 Grill (broil) for 2–3 minutes until sizzling. Top each with a little crème fraîche and cheese and return to the grill just until bubbling.

4 Serve straight away with oatcakes.

Baked Crusted Avocado with Prawns

Avocado with prawns is a dish rich in phosphorus, zinc and vitamin A. Use individual gratin dishes instead of the shells, if you prefer.

SERVES 4

2 ripe avocados, halved and stoned (pitted)

5 ml/1 tsp lemon juice

175 g/6 oz cooked peeled prawns (shrimp)

100 g/4 oz/½ cup low-fat soft cheese

45 ml/3 tbsp low-fat mayonnaise

15 ml/1 tbsp tomato purée (paste)

A few drops of Tabasco sauce

A few drops of Worcestershire sauce

25 g/1 oz/2 tbsp low-fat sunflower, soya or olive oil spread

50g/2 oz/1 cup fresh wholemeal breadcrumbs

25 g/1 oz/¼ cup freshly grated Parmesan cheese

Wedges of lemon and sprigs of parsley, for garnishing

To serve:

Wholemeal toast

1   Preheat the oven to 200°C/400°F/gas 6/fan oven 180°C.

2   Scoop the avocado flesh into a bowl. Reserve the shells. Toss the avocado with the lemon juice and prawns.

3   Mix the cheese, mayonnaise, tomato purée and sauces, then mix with the avocado.

4   Spoon the mixture back into the shells and place in shallow individual ovenproof dishes. Melt the low-fat spread and mix with the breadcrumbs and Parmesan cheese. Scatter this mixture over the filling.

5   Bake for 10–15 minutes until the tops are golden and the filling piping hot. Serve straight away.

Italian Scrambled Eggs with Tomatoes, Peppers and Olives

This is a version of the classic dish, piperade, but with the addition of olives for added vitality. The peppers are rich in vitamin C, which will help keep you fit, healthy and alert. This dish makes a great light meal any time of day.

SERVES 4

30 ml/2 tbsp olive oil

25 g/1 oz/2 tbsp low-fat sunflower, soya or olive oil spread

2 large onions, halved and sliced

1 green (bell) pepper, sliced

1 red pepper, sliced

1 yellow pepper, sliced

4 ripe tomatoes, roughly chopped

1 garlic clove, crushed

8 stoned (pitted) black olives, sliced

6 eggs, beaten

30 ml/2 tbsp water

Salt and freshly ground black pepper

To serve:

Hot wholemeal toast

1 Heat the oil and low-fat spread in a large frying pan (skillet) over a fairly high heat.

2 Add the onions, peppers, tomatoes and garlic and cook, stirring, for 5 minutes until soft.

3 Add the olives, eggs, just a pinch of salt and lots of pepper and cook over a gentle heat, stirring until scrambled.

4 Serve straight away with hot toast.

Mushroom and Leek Quiche

Wholemeal pastry, made with cholesterol-lowering low-fat polyunsaturated or monounsaturated spread, is a good source of complex carbohydrates. Filled with a mixture of mushrooms and leeks in a cheese custard, it makes an ideal lunch to keep you sustained all afternoon.

SERVES 4

For the pastry (paste):

175 g/6 oz/1½ cups plain (all-purpose) wholemeal flour, plus extra for dusting

1.5 ml/¼ tsp celery salt

75 g/3 oz/⅓ cup low-fat sunflower, soya or olive oil spread

60–75 ml/4–5 tbsp cold water

For the filling:

100 g/4 oz button mushrooms, sliced

1 leek, trimmed and thinly sliced

15 ml/1 tbsp sunflower or olive oil

2.5 ml/½ tsp dried oregano

50 g/2 oz/½ cup grated low-fat Cheddar cheese

Salt and freshly ground black pepper

300 ml/½ pt/1¼ cups milk

2 eggs

To serve:

A green salad

1 Make the pastry. Put the flour and celery salt in a bowl. Add the low-fat spread and work in with a fork until the mixture resembles breadcrumbs. Mix with enough cold water to form a firm dough. Roll out on a lightly floured surface and use to line a 20 cm/8 in flan dish (pie pan). Prick the base with a fork. Place on a baking (cookie) sheet.

2 Preheat the oven to 190°C/375°F/gas 5/fan oven 170°C. Fry (sauté) the mushrooms and leek in the oil for 3 minutes, stirring occasionally, until softened.

3 Turn into the flan case (pie shell). Top with the cheese and sprinkle with oregano.

4 Beat the milk and eggs together and season lightly.

5 Pour into the flan case and bake in the oven for about 30 minutes until the filling is set and golden brown.

6 Serve hot or cold with a green salad.

Cheese Soufflé

Making a soufflé normally involves making a thick sauce first. My version simply mixes the ingredients together – so the preparation couldn't be simpler and there is no nasty saucepan to clean up. Cheese and eggs will give you lots of the nutrients you require to fight fatigue and cooked this way they aren't heavy on the stomach either!

SERVES 4

A little low-fat sunflower, soya or olive oil spread, for greasing

100 g/4 oz/$\frac{1}{2}$ cup finely grated low-fat Cheddar cheese

30 ml/2 tbsp milk

15 g/$\frac{1}{2}$ oz/2 tbsp plain (all-purpose) flour

1.5 ml/$\frac{1}{4}$ tsp made English mustard

30 ml/2 tbsp freshly grated Parmesan cheese

A pinch of salt

A good grinding of black pepper

2 eggs, separated

To serve:

A tomato salad

1 Preheat the oven to 190°C/375°F/gas 5/fan oven 170°C. Grease a 15 cm/6 in soufflé dish.

2 Put all the ingredients except the egg whites in a bowl and mix with a wooden spoon until well blended.

3 Whisk the egg whites until stiff and fold gently into the mixture with a metal spoon.

4 Turn into the prepared dish and bake in the oven for about 25 minutes until well risen, golden and just set.

5 Serve straight away with a tomato salad.

Tuna Mornay on Spinach

Fish is an important part of a healthy fatigue-fighting regime. Canned tuna is a good choice, being so cheap and widely available. I prefer it canned in water rather than oil or brine, to avoid excess fat or sodium. Mixed with spinach and cheese, it is an ideal lunch combination.

SERVES 2–4

---

40 g/1½ oz/3 tbsp low-fat sunflower, soya or olive oil spread

2 onions, thinly sliced

20 g/³⁄₄ oz/3 tbsp plain (all-purpose) flour

300 ml/½ pt/1¼ cups milk

Salt and freshly ground black pepper

75 g/3 oz/³⁄₄ cup grated low-fat Cheddar cheese

225 g/8 oz frozen leaf spinach, thawed

1 × 185 g/6½ oz/small can of tuna, drained

To serve:

Hot wholemeal toast

1 Melt the low-fat spread in a saucepan over a fairly high heat. Add the onions and cook, stirring, for 3 minutes until softened.

2 Stir the flour into the pan and cook for 1 minute. Remove from the heat and gradually stir in the milk. Return to the heat, bring to the boil and cook for 2 minutes, stirring.

3 Preheat the oven to 190°C/375°F/gas 5/fan oven 170°C.

4 Squeeze the spinach well to drain off excess liquid. Spread out in a fairly shallow ovenproof dish. Spread the drained tuna over the top. Pour the sauce over and sprinkle with the remaining cheese.

5 Bake in the oven for about 30 minutes until golden, bubbling and hot through.

6 Serve with hot wholemeal toast.

SUPER SNACK LUNCHES

You may not want – or be able – to cook at midday. But that doesn't mean that you can't have a delicious, nutritious lunch. All the recipes in this section are designed to tempt your taste buds and keep you functioning at your best all afternoon. Most of them are ideal for lunchboxes and can be prepared in advance, perhaps even the night before, if you are super-organised!

Tuna and Haricot Open Sandwiches

The perfect combination of vitamins, minerals, protein and complex carbohydrates, all in a bite! If you aren't going to eat them straight away, make the tuna mixture and keep the crispbreads separate, to spread when you're ready to eat, or they'll go soggy.

SERVES 4

1 × 425 g/15 oz/large can of haricot (navy) beans, drained

1 garlic clove, crushed

1 × 85 g/3½ oz/very small can of tuna, drained

30 ml/2 tbsp sunflower oil

15 ml/1 tbsp lemon juice

A good pinch of cayenne

8 rye crispbreads

A little low-fat sunflower, soya or olive oil spread

15 ml/1 tbsp chopped fresh parsley

To serve:

Slices of cucumber and tomato

1 Put all the ingredients except the crispbreads, low-fat spread and parsley in a blender or food processor and run the machine until smooth, stopping and scraping down the sides, if necessary.

2 Seal the mixture in an airtight container until ready to use.

3 When ready to eat, put a scraping of low-fat spread on the crispbreads. Pile the tuna mixture on top and sprinkle with parsley.

4 Serve with slices of cucumber and tomato on the side.

Smoked Mackerel and Pink Grapefruit Club Sandwiches

This is a divine combination and packed with vitality ingredients. Elegant and sophisticated, it is one of the tastiest club sandwiches I have ever created.

SERVES 4

1 pink grapefruit

2 large or 4 small smoked mackerel fillets

Freshly ground black pepper

12 slices of granary bread

A little low-fat sunflower, soya or olive oil spread

100 g/4 oz/$\frac{1}{2}$ cup low-fat soft cheese

25 g/1 oz lambs' tongue lettuce

1 Cut all the peel and pith off the grapefruit, then chop the flesh. Discard any very tough membranes. Drain on kitchen paper (paper towels).

2 Skin and flake the mackerel, discarding any bones. Season with pepper.

3 Toast the bread. Put a scraping of low-fat spread on eight slices. Top the remainder with the soft cheese.

4 Top four slices of the 'buttered' toast with the mackerel. Cover with the cheese-topped toast, then spread with the grapefruit and top with the lettuce. Top with the final slices of toast, 'buttered' sides down.

5 Cut the sandwiches into halves and secure each half with a cocktail stick (toothpick).

Curried Chicken, Mango and Coriander Naan Toppers

Naan breads make the perfect complex carbohydrate vehicle for a lunchtime snack. Here they are topped with chicken and fresh mango in a low-fat dressing. You could also try seafood or diced cheese instead of the chicken.

SERVES 4

---

1 small fresh mango, peeled

45 ml/3 tbsp low-fat mayonnaise

10 ml/2 tsp curry paste

100 g/4 oz cooked chicken, chopped, discarding any skin

30 ml/2 tbsp chopped fresh coriander (cilantro)

Freshly ground black pepper

4 small plain naan breads, warmed if liked

15 ml/1 tbsp toasted flaked (slivered) almonds

1 Cut all the flesh off the mango and chop.

2 Mix the mayonnaise with the curry paste. Stir in the chicken, mango and coriander. Season to taste with pepper.

3 Pile on top of the naans.

4 Scatter the almonds over and serve.

Chinese Chicken Wraps

Do not heat the filling ingredients if you are taking these as a packed lunch – they taste just as good cold. The tortillas provide slow-release carbohydrates, the vegetables and seeds give you plenty of fatigue-fighting nutrients and the chicken contains the small amount of protein you need.

SERVES 4

100 g/4 oz cooked chicken, skinned and cut into neat pieces

1 × 425 g/15 oz/large can of stir-fry vegetables, rinsed and drained

15 ml/1 tbsp black bean sauce

15 ml/1 tbsp toasted sesame seeds

4 large flour tortillas

1 Put the chicken, vegetables and black bean sauce in a saucepan and heat through until piping hot, stirring all the time.

2 Sprinkle in the sesame seeds.

3 Warm the tortillas briefly in the microwave, if liked.

4 Divide the chicken mixture into four. Pile a portion on one quarter of each tortilla, fold the tortilla in half, then quarters, over the filling, to form a cone filled with the Chinese chicken mixture.

Prawn and Artichoke Mega Sandwiches

Prawns are packed full of phosphorus and zinc. Served with canned artichokes and carrots (for added vitality) in thick, wholegrain bread, you have a winning combination that will keep you fresh and sustained right through till teatime.

SERVES 4

A little low-fat sunflower, soya or olive oil spread

8 thick slices of granary bread

100 g/4 oz cooked peeled prawns (shrimp), thawed if frozen

1 × 425 g/15 oz/large can of artichoke hearts, drained

45 ml/3 tbsp low-fat crème fraîche

1 carrot, grated

Freshly ground black pepper

4 round lettuce leaves

1 Put a scraping of low-fat spread on the bread.

2 Drain the prawns and artichokes well on kitchen paper (paper towels). Tip the prawns into a bowl. Chop the artichoke hearts and add to the bowl.

3 Mix in the crème fraîche and carrot and season well with pepper.

4 Top each of four slices of bread with a lettuce leaf, breaking the thick stalks if necessary so the leaves lie flat.

5 Top with the prawn mixture, then the other slices of bread. Press down lightly and cut into triangles.

Cold Chilli Bean and Tuna Rolls

Tuna and beans are both great fatigue-fighters. Here they are wrapped in flour tortillas for slow-release energy and blended with peppers and tomatoes to make parcels packed with vitamin C.

SERVES 4

1 × 425 g/15 oz/large can of red kidney beans, drained

1 × 185 g/6½ oz/small can of tuna, drained

5 ml/1 tsp clear honey

1 green (bell) pepper, chopped

2.5 cm/1 in piece of cucumber, chopped

2 tomatoes, chopped

Salt and freshly ground black pepper

A few drops of hot chilli sauce, to taste

4 large or 8 small flour tortillas

1 wedge of iceberg lettuce, shredded

60 ml/4 tbsp low-fat crème fraîche

1 Mash the beans and stir in all the remaining ingredients except the tortillas, lettuce and crème fraîche.

2 Spread the tortillas with the bean and tuna mixture.

3 Top each with the lettuce, then the crème fraîche, then roll up tightly.

Cheese Blushers

These are bursting with vitamin B for a great brightness boost to keep you performing at your best all afternoon. Bagels add the sustained energy component and the overall effect is one of tasty indulgence!

SERVES 4

---

45 ml/3 tbsp low-fat mayonnaise

100 g/4 oz/1 cup crumbled Feta cheese

1 small red onion, finely chopped

2 cooked baby beetroot (red beets), drained and diced

Freshly ground black pepper

4 bagels, split

A little low-fat sunflower, soya or olive oil spread

8 slices of cucumber, for garnishing

1 Mix together all the ingredients except the bagels and low-fat spread.

2 Toast the bagels, if liked, and spread with just a scraping of low-fat spread.

3 Pile the cheese mixture on top and garnish with a twist of cucumber on each.

Grilled Sardine and Horseradish Snack

Oily fish is vital for fatigue-fighters. Canned sardines are a terrific example, but despite being highly nutritious and inexpensive, they're probably one of the most overlooked ingredients on the supermarket shelves. Blended with a touch of horseradish, they make a mouth-watering snack meal.

SERVES 4

4 thick slices of wholemeal bread

15 g/½ oz/1 tbsp low-fat sunflower, soya or olive oil spread

10 ml/2 tsp horseradish relish

2 × 120 g/4½ oz/small cans of sardines in oil, drained

1 beefsteak tomato

Lemon juice

Freshly ground black pepper

15 ml/1 tbsp chopped fresh parsley

1 Preheat the grill (broiler) and toast the bread on both sides.

2 Mash the low-fat spread with the horseradish in a small bowl.

3 Mash the sardines, including the bones – they are calcium-rich and very good for you. Stir into the horseradish mixture.

4 Cut the tomato into four thick slices, discarding the ends. Top the toast with the tomato slices and grill (broil) for 1 minute.

5 Pile the sardine mixture on top. Sprinkle with lemon juice and pepper. Grill for about 3 minutes until sizzling.

6 Sprinkle with parsley and eat straight away.

Hot Salmon and Celery Toasties

Salmon may be more expensive than tuna but pink salmon is still relatively cheap. Here it is mixed with crunchy celery, a few chopped cornichons and some naturally low-fat Edam cheese, for a hot snack to fill you up but keep you alert. Eat the bones, too, for added calcium.

SERVES 2–4

1 × 200 g/7 oz/small can of pink or red salmon

30 ml/2 tbsp low-fat mayonnaise

4 cornichons, chopped

1 celery stick, finely chopped

A squeeze of lemon juice

4 thick slices of wholemeal bread

A little low-fat sunflower, soya or olive oil spread

50 g/2 oz/½ cup grated Edam cheese

Freshly ground black pepper

1 Drain the fish, discard any skin and mash well. You can remove the bones if you like but I do recommend you eat them, as they are very good for you!

2 Mix in the mayonnaise, cornichons and celery.

3 Preheat the grill (broiler) and toast the bread on both sides. Leave on the grill rack. Spread one side with just a scraping of low-fat spread, then top with the salmon mixture. Sprinkle the cheese over and add a good grinding of pepper.

4 Grill (broil) under a moderate heat until the cheese melts and bubbles and the topping is hot through.

5 Serve straight away.

Quick Pan Pizza

This one isn't suitable for a lunchbox, but it does make a great, quick, fatigue-fighting meal any time. Add other toppings of your choice before adding the cheese, if you like.

SERVES 2
---

100 g/4 oz/1 cup self-raising (self-rising) wholemeal flour

A pinch of salt

45 ml/3 tbsp sunflower or olive oil

45 ml/3 tbsp tomato purée (paste)

1.5 ml/¼ tsp dried oregano

75 g/3 oz/¾ cup grated low-fat Mozzarella cheese

2 tomatoes, sliced

2 stoned (pitted) black or green olives, sliced

A few fresh basil leaves, torn

1 Mix the flour and salt in a bowl. Add 30 ml/2 tbsp of the oil and mix with enough cold water to form a soft but not sticky dough.

2 Knead gently on a lightly floured surface and roll out to a round the size of a medium frying pan (skillet).

3 Heat the remaining oil in a frying pan and add the round of dough. Cook for 3 minutes until golden brown underneath.

4 Turn over and spread with the tomato purée, oregano and cheese. Lay the tomato slices on top and sprinkle with the olives and basil leaves. Cover with a lid or foil and cook for 2–3 minutes.

5 Meanwhile, preheat the grill (broiler).

6 Remove the cover from the pan and transfer the pan to the grill. Cook for 2–3 minutes or until the cheese melts and bubbles.

7 Serve hot.

Quick Tuna Noodles

This is really a healthy version of that great student standby: 'pot noodle'. It takes only minutes to make using the almost instant-cook Chinese egg noodles. Tuna and sweetcorn are always a great combination and they have all the stamina-building nutrients you need.

SERVES 2

---

2 slabs of Chinese egg noodles

1 × 200 g/7 oz/small can of sweetcorn (corn), drained

1 × 185 g/6½ oz/small can of tuna, drained

60 ml/4 tbsp low-fat mayonnaise

25 g/1 oz/¼ cup grated low-fat Cheddar cheese

Freshly ground black pepper

1 Put the noodles in a saucepan. Cover with boiling water, bring back to the boil, turn off the heat and leave to stand for 5 minutes, stirring once or twice.

2 Drain thoroughly and return to the pan.

3 Add the sweetcorn, tuna, mayonnaise and cheese and toss over a low heat until well mixed and hot through. Season with pepper.

4 Spoon into bowls and serve.

Fast Food Lunches

There isn't always time to be creative, so this list provides a few ideas for energising fast food to grab at lunchtime. Avoid sugary and fizzy drinks – choose pure fruit juice or water.

- Wholemeal sandwich or wrap filled with salad and egg, tuna, prawns or chicken; an apple or orange
- Cheese, wholegrain crackers, tomatoes and a chunk of cucumber; a small packet of mixed nuts and raisins
- Bagel filled with low-fat soft cheese, a spoonful of pesto, sliced tomato and rocket; a small packet of ready-to-eat dried apricots
- Cold chicken portion – 1 breast or 2 drumsticks – plus a wholegrain roll with salad; a banana and a small carton of low-fat, sugar-free yoghurt
- Pasta or rice salad with seafood, cheese or chicken and diced salad vegetables, in low-fat dressing; a nectarine or peach
- Baked beans (reduced-sugar, low-salt) on wholemeal toast with a little grated cheese; 2 satsumas
- A tub of plain or flavoured cottage cheese with sticks of raw vegetables, such as carrots, celery, courgettes (zucchini) and (bell) peppers; a small bag of ready-to-eat dried tropical fruit mix
- Sliced rollmop herrings, with diced cucumber, potato salad (with low-fat mayonnaise) and a rye crispbread; a pear or an apple
- Cold, lean, roast beef in a wholegrain sandwich with a scraping of horseradish, low-fat mayonnaise and lettuce; a carton of low-fat, sugar-free fromage frais with fresh raspberries or strawberries
- $\frac{1}{2}$ small round ogen, cantaloupe or galia melon filled with prawns or tuna tossed in a dash of olive oil and lemon juice, with a multigrain roll with soft cheese and chives; a small bag of raw cashew nuts or peanuts
- A small tub of low-fat hummus or taramasalata with raw vegetable sticks and 1 small wholemeal pitta bread; 2 plums

MEAT MAIN MEALS

It's good to know that lean red meat helps fight fatigue – it makes a change from all the bad press it's had in recent years! Just make sure that you trim off all excess fat before cooking.

Steak Strips and Spinach Sizzle with Crunchy Almond Ribbons

I usually use wholewheat tagliatelle but you may have to go to a health food shop to find this. So, if you decide to use ordinary white noodles, don't worry – they are a good source of complex carbohydrates and there are plenty of other fatigue-fighting nutrients in this dish without the added fibre.

SERVES 4

350 g/12 oz beef stir-fry meat

Finely grated zest and juice of 1 orange

225 g/8 oz thin ribbon noodles

30 ml/2 tbsp sunflower oil

1 large onion, finely chopped

100 g/4 oz button mushrooms, sliced

450 g/1 lb baby spinach

15 ml/1 tbsp light soy sauce

30 ml/2 tbsp Worcestershire sauce

30 ml/2 tbsp water

25 g/1 oz/2 tbsp low-fat sunflower, soya or olive oil spread

25 g/1 oz/½ cup fresh wholemeal breadcrumbs

25 g/1 oz/¼ cup chopped almonds

1 Place the beef in a shallow dish and toss in the orange zest and juice. Leave to stand for at least 2 hours.

2 Cook the noodles according to the packet directions. Drain in a colander.

3 Meanwhile, heat the oil in a large frying pan (skillet) or wok over a moderate heat. Add the onion and cook, stirring, for 2 minutes to soften.

4 Add the beef and mushrooms and toss for 3 minutes.

5 Add the spinach, soy and Worcestershire sauces and the water. Toss for 1 minute.

6 Melt the low-fat spread in a large saucepan and add the breadcrumbs and nuts. Toss over a fairly high heat until golden. Add the cooked noodles to the pan and toss to coat, then reheat.

7 Pile the noodles on warm plates. Top with the beef mixture and serve.

Beef Stroganoff
with Green Peppercorns

*Luxurious, elegant and highly nutritious – this has to be the
perfect combination for a meal to impress friends or family.
The dash of brandy won't cause drowsiness because the
alcohol evaporates when it is flamed.*

SERVES 4

---

225 g/8 oz/1 cup wild rice mix

100 g/4 oz French (green) beans, cut into short lengths

2 large onions, sliced

25 g/1 oz/2 tbsp low-fat sunflower, soya or olive oil spread

450 g/1 lb beef stir-fry meat

100 g/4 oz button mushrooms, sliced

30 ml/2 tbsp brandy

15 ml/1 tbsp pickled green peppercorns

300 ml/½ pt/1¼ cups low-fat crème fraîche

Salt and freshly ground black pepper

30 ml/2 tbsp chopped fresh parsley

To serve:

A green salad

1 Cook the wild rice mix according to the packet
   directions, adding the beans for the last 4 minutes'
   cooking time. Drain and keep warm.

2 Meanwhile, fry (sauté) the onions in the low-fat spread
   in a large frying pan (skillet) for 3 minutes, stirring
   until lightly golden.

3 Add the beef and mushrooms and fry for a further
   2 minutes, stirring all the time.

4 Add the brandy and ignite. Shake the pan until the
   flames subside.

5 Stir in the peppercorns, crème fraîche and seasoning to taste. Reheat but do not allow to boil.

6 Pile the rice mix on to warm plates and spoon the stroganoff to one side. Garnish with chopped parsley and serve with a green salad.

Chilli con Carne
with Guacamole on Rice

A classic dish with a modern approach – this version is low in fat but high in vitality-inducing nutrients. It is guaranteed to fill you up and should keep your blood-sugar levels up for several hours. Serve it with a green salad.

SERVES 4

225 g/8 oz extra-lean minced (ground) lamb or beef

1 large onion, chopped

2.5 ml/¹/₂ tsp chilli powder

5 ml/1 tsp ground cumin

5 ml/1 tsp dried oregano

450 ml/³/₄ pt/2 cups passata (sieved tomatoes)

2 × 425 g/15 oz/large cans of red kidney beans, drained

15 ml/1 tbsp tomato purée (paste)

5 ml/1 tsp clear honey

Salt and freshly ground black pepper

225 g/8 oz/1 cup long-grain rice

For the guacamole:

2 ripe avocados

Juice of 1 lime

A few drops each of Worcestershire and Tabasco sauce

30 ml/2 tbsp sunflower oil

2 tomatoes, skinned, seeded and chopped

5 cm/2 in piece of cucumber, finely chopped

1 Put the meat and onion in a saucepan and dry-fry, stirring, over a high heat for 5 minutes until the meat is no longer pink and all the grains are separate.

2 Stir the chilli powder, cumin and oregano into the meat and cook for a further 1 minute.

3 Stir in the passata, beans, tomato purée, honey and a little salt and pepper.

4 Bring to the boil, turn down the heat and simmer for 20 minutes, stirring occasionally.

5 Meanwhile, cook the rice in plenty of boiling, lightly salted water for 10 minutes or according to the packet directions. Drain, rinse with boiling water and drain again.

6 Make the guacamole. Halve the avocados, remove the stones (pits) and scoop the flesh into a bowl. Mash in the lime juice, then beat in the sauces and sunflower oil. Finally, stir in the tomato and cucumber and season lightly.

7 Spoon the rice into large warm bowls. Top with the meat mixture and garnish with a large spoonful of guacamole.

Greek-style Stuffed Aubergines

Aubergines make the perfect vehicle for other health-giving nutrients – here in the form of red meat, olives, garlic and concentrated tomato. When served with wholemeal pittas and a mixed salad, this is a perfectly balanced meal.

SERVES 4

2 large aubergines (eggplants)

1 onion, finely chopped

1 garlic clove, crushed

175 g/6 oz extra-lean minced (ground) steak

30 ml/2 tbsp tomato purée (paste)

1.5 ml/¼ tsp ground cinnamon

2.5 ml/½ tsp dried oregano

12 stoned (pitted) black olives, sliced

30 ml/2 tbsp water

2.5 ml/½ tsp clear honey

Freshly ground black pepper

200 g/7 oz/1¾ cups crumbled Feta cheese

30 ml/2 tbsp chopped fresh parsley

To serve:

A mixed salad and warm wholemeal pitta breads

1   Halve the aubergines lengthways. Cook in boiling water for 5 minutes or until almost tender. Drain, rinse with cold water and drain again. Scoop out most of the aubergine with a teaspoon, leaving a wall all round. Chop the scooped-out flesh.

2   Preheat the oven to 190°C/375°F/gas 5/fan oven 170°C. Put the onion, garlic and meat in a saucepan and cook, stirring all the time, until the beef is no longer pink and all the grains are separate. Stir in the chopped aubergine, tomato purée, cinnamon, oregano, olives, water, honey and pepper to taste.

3 Put the aubergine shells in a roasting tin (pan) and fill with the meat mixture.

4 Sprinkle with the cheese. Add 60 ml/4 tbsp of water to the tin and cover the tin with foil.

5 Bake in the oven for about 35 minutes until the aubergines are tender and cooked through and the cheese has melted.

6 Transfer to warm plates and sprinkle with parsley.

7 Serve with a mixed salad and warm wholemeal pitta breads.

Minted Lamb Tagine
with Pears and Raisins

*Red meat, fruits and vegetables, all generously piled on a bed
of couscous: this is a delicious dish, packed with flavour.
Enjoy it knowing you'll feel full but not blown out, and
definitely wide awake!*

SERVES 4

---

450 g/1 lb diced lean stewing lamb

*1 bunch of spring onions (scallions),
cut into short lengths*

2 carrots, diced

1 large garlic clove, crushed

1.5 ml/¼ tsp ground cinnamon

1.5 ml/¼ tsp ground ginger

Salt and freshly ground black pepper

*900 ml/1½ pts/3¾ cups lamb stock,
made with 2 stock cubes*

10 ml/2 tsp tomato purée (paste)

*100 g/4 oz/⅔ cup ready-to-eat dried pears,
cut into chunks*

50 g/2 oz/⅓ cup raisins

2 courgettes (zucchini), diced

1 green (bell) pepper, diced

225 g/8 oz/1⅓ cups couscous

30 ml/2 tbsp chopped fresh parsley

30 ml/2 tbsp chopped fresh mint

---

1 Put the lamb, onions and carrots in a large saucepan
with the garlic, spices, a little salt and pepper and the
lamb stock. Bring to the boil, stirring. Reduce the heat,
part-cover and cook gently for 1½ hours, stirring
occasionally.

2 Put the couscous in a bowl and add just enough boiling water to cover. Leave to stand for 5 minutes, then tip into a steamer or metal colander.

3 Add the fruits and vegetables to the lamb mixture with half the herbs. Sit the steamer of couscous on top of the saucepan, cover and cook for a further 15 minutes.

4 Fluff up the couscous with a fork. If necessary, boil the tagine rapidly without a lid, stirring all the time, to reduce the liquid to a thick sauce. Taste and adjust the seasoning.

5 Spoon the couscous on to plates. Spoon the lamb mixture on top.

6 Serve sprinkled with the remaining parsley and mint.

Seekh Kebabs
with Fresh Mango Salsa

The fresh mango salsa sets off the richness and delicate spiciness of the meat. It also adds loads of fatigue-fighting nutrients to the dish.

SERVES 4

---

1 onion, grated

15 ml/1 tbsp grated fresh root ginger

5 ml/1 tsp ground cinnamon

5 ml/1 tsp ground cumin

2.5 ml/¹/₂ tsp chilli powder

450 g/1 lb extra-lean minced (ground) lamb

Juice of ¹/₂ lime

30 ml/2 tbsp Greek-style plain low-fat yoghurt

*30 ml/2 tbsp plain (all-purpose) flour,
plus extra for dusting*

30 ml/2 tbsp chopped fresh coriander (cilantro)

2.5 ml/¹/₂ tsp salt

Freshly ground black pepper

For the salsa:

*1 large ripe mango, peeled, stoned (pitted)
and roughly chopped*

150 ml/¹/₄ pt/²/₃ cup Greek-style plain low-fat yoghurt

15 ml/1 tbsp chopped fresh mint

15 ml/1 tbsp chopped fresh parsley

Juice of ¹/₂ lime

Wedges of lime, for garnishing

To serve:

Tabbouleh (see page 154) and lettuce leaves

1 Put the onion in a large bowl with the spices and mix to a paste.

2 Add the lamb, lime juice, yoghurt, flour, coriander and salt and pepper. Mix well with your hands to combine.

3 Preheat the grill (broiler).

4 With floured hands, divide the mixture into eight pieces and shape each piece into a sausage shape around a skewer. Lay on foil on a grill rack. Grill (broil) for about 10 minutes, turning once, until golden brown and cooked through.

5 Mix all the salsa ingredients together.

6 Slide the kebabs off the skewers on to plates and garnish with wedges of lime. Put a lettuce leaf on each plate and pile some tabbouleh inside.

7 Serve with the salsa.

Red-cooked Lamb
with Green Thai Rice

Another Asian favourite of mine. I prefer to buy a half leg of lamb and dice it myself but any diced lamb that is free from fat is fine. The green rice is rich in iron and folate, and also provides slow-release carbohydrate to keep your energy levels up.

SERVES 4–6

---

700 g/1½ lb lean diced lamb

2 large garlic cloves, chopped

1 bunch of spring onions (scallions), cut into short lengths

1 × 200 g/7 oz/small can of pimientos, drained

For the red sauce:

2.5 cm/1 in piece of fresh root ginger, peeled and grated

5 ml/1 tsp Chinese five-spice powder

15 ml/1 tbsp tomato purée (paste)

30 ml/2 tbsp dry sherry or pure apple juice

60 ml/4 tbsp light soy sauce

450 ml/¾ pt/2 cups beef stock, made with 1 stock cube

10 ml/2 tsp clear honey

For the green rice:

225 g/8 oz/1 cup Thai fragrant rice

15 g/½ oz/1 tbsp low-fat sunflower, soya or olive oil spread

1 bunch of watercress, trimmed and chopped

15 ml/1 tbsp chopped fresh coriander (cilantro)

15 ml/1 tbsp chopped fresh parsley

Sprigs of parsley or coriander, for garnishing

1 Put the lamb, garlic and spring onions in a flameproof casserole (Dutch oven). Cut eight thin strips off the pimientos and reserve. Chop the remainder and add to the lamb.

2 Mix the red sauce ingredients together and pour over. Stir well.

3 Cook over a high heat until boiling. Turn down the heat until just gently bubbling round the edges. Stir again, cover with a lid and cook for 1½ hours.

4 Remove the lid, turn up the heat and cook rapidly for a few minutes, stirring all the time, until the sauce is rich and thick.

5 Meanwhile, cook the rice according to the packet directions. Drain.

6 Rinse out the saucepan and melt the low-fat spread in it. Stir in the watercress and chopped herbs and cook, tossing, for 30 seconds. Return the rice to the pan and stir well until thoroughly mixed and slightly sticky. Season to taste.

7 Spoon on to warm plates and top with the lamb. Garnish each serving with two strips of pimiento in a cross on top of the lamb and sprigs of parsley or coriander to one side.

Lamb Steaks with Mint Jus and Leek and Parsnip Mash

Parsnips, potatoes and leeks blend beautifully in this energy-giving mash. When topped with lean lamb and a lovely mint-flavoured gravy, it is a delicious, revitalising meal.

SERVES 4

---

2 large potatoes

2 large parsnips

2 large leeks

40 g/1½ oz/3 tbsp low-fat sunflower, soya or olive oil spread

4 lamb steaks, trimmed of any fat

Salt and freshly ground black pepper

15 ml/1 tbsp cornflour (cornstarch)

15 ml/1 tbsp bottled garden mint

2.5 ml/½ tsp clear honey

To serve:

Broccoli and baby carrots

1 Peel and cut the potatoes and parsnips into small, even-sized chunks. Place in a pan, cover with cold, lightly salted water and bring to the boil.

2 Trim the leeks, slice each one almost right through lengthways, from the green end to the white, and wash well under running water. Cut into chunks and add to the potatoes and parsnips.

3 Bring back to the boil, reduce the heat, part-cover and simmer for about 10 minutes or until the vegetables are tender. Drain, reserving the cooking liquid.

4 Mash the boiled vegetables with half the low-fat spread and keep warm.

5 Meanwhile, melt the remaining spread and brush over both sides of the lamb steaks. Season lightly.

6 Place on foil on the grill (broiler) rack and grill (broil) for 5–8 minutes on each side until cooked to your liking. Transfer to a serving plate and keep warm.

7 Tip the cooking juices from the foil into a small saucepan and scrape any sediment off the foil. Stir in the cornflour and garden mint. Measure 300 ml/ ½ pt/1¼ cups of the vegetable cooking water into the pan and stir to blend completely. Add the honey. Bring to the boil, and cook for 1 minute, stirring all the time. Season to taste.

8 Spoon the mashed vegetables on to four warm plates. Rest a lamb steak against each pile. Spoon the mint jus over and serve with broccoli and baby carrots.

Pork and Bean Hotpot

Continental sausages are high in fat so I don't recommend you eat much of them. However, using a small amount in a recipe like this imparts a fabulous flavour without being detrimental to your fatigue-fighting! There is no point in using canned, ready-cooked beans for this dish as it is best slow-cooked for a very long period.

SERVES 4

---

225 g/8 oz/1½ cups dried haricot (navy) beans, soaked in cold water overnight

450 ml/¾ pt/2 cups water

1 beef stock cube

15 ml/1 tbsp olive oil

225 g/8 oz lean diced pork

1 large onion, chopped

2 carrots, diced

2 celery sticks, chopped

½ small swede (rutabaga), diced

50 g/2 oz diced chorizo sausage

1 × 400 g/14 oz/large can of chopped tomatoes

10 ml/2 tsp clear honey

2.5 ml/½ tsp dried sage

Salt and freshly ground black pepper

30 ml/2 tbsp snipped fresh chives, for garnishing

To serve:

Crusty wholemeal bread

1 Preheat the oven to 150°C/300°F/gas 2/fan oven 135°C.

2 Drain the soaked beans and place in a large, flameproof casserole (Dutch oven) with the water. Bring to the boil over a high heat and boil rapidly for 10 minutes.

3 Crumble in the stock cube and stir until dissolved.

4 Heat the oil in a frying pan (skillet) over a high heat. Fry (sauté) the pork, onion, carrots, celery and swede for 2 minutes, stirring.

5 Add to the casserole with the remaining ingredients, stir and bring the mixture back to the boil.

6 Cover and place in the oven for 4 hours or until the beans are really tender and bathed in a rich sauce.

7 Taste and re-season, if necessary. Sprinkle with chives and serve with crusty wholemeal bread.

Liver, Onion and Apple Hotpot with Crushed Leeks and Broad Beans

Liver contains high levels of iron, and the fruit and vegetables have lots of vitalising nutrients – this really makes the perfect meal, especially as it is topped with golden sliced potatoes for added slow-release energy.

SERVES 4

---

450 g/1 lb pigs' liver, cut into bite-sized pieces

30 ml/2 tbsp milk

40 g/1½ oz/3 tbsp low-fat sunflower, soya or olive oil spread

3 large onions, sliced

2 large carrots, thinly sliced

2 eating (dessert) apples, sliced

15 ml/1 tbsp plain (all-purpose) flour

450 ml/¾ pt/2 cups beef stock, made with 1 stock cube

5 ml/1 tsp dried sage

Salt and freshly ground black pepper

450 g/1 lb potatoes, scrubbed and sliced

2 large leeks, thinly sliced

350 g/12 oz fresh shelled or frozen broad (fava) beans

30 ml/2 tbsp snipped fresh chives

---

1 Preheat the oven to 190°C/375°F/gas 5/fan oven 170°C.

2 Soak the liver in the milk for 15 minutes. Drain.

3 Heat 15 g/½ oz/1 tbsp of the low-fat spread in a flameproof casserole (Dutch oven) over a fairly high heat. Fry (sauté) the onions and carrots for 3 minutes, stirring, until lightly golden. Add the liver and fry for 2 minutes.

4 Stir in the apples, flour, stock and sage. Bring to the boil, stirring. Season to taste.

5 Lay the potatoes over the top and dot with half of the remaining spread.

6 Cover the casserole with a lid or foil and bake in the oven for 30 minutes. Remove the lid or foil and continue to cook for a further 30 minutes or until cooked through and the top is turning golden brown.

7 Meanwhile, cook the leeks and broad beans in boiling, lightly salted water for 6–8 minutes or until tender. Drain and return to the pan. Add the remaining spread. Roughly crush with a potato masher over a gentle heat, then stir in the chives.

8 Spoon the hot pot on to warm plates and serve with the crushed leeks and beans.

Fragrant Wholewheat Spaghetti with Cherry Tomatoes, Pork and Onions

You can use minced roast pork if you want to use up the leftovers on a Monday. I like to use wholewheat spaghetti in this: it provides added fibre and offsets the richness of the meat and onions but you can use white pasta if you prefer. Make sure you serve it with the green salad for the added nutrients.

SERVES 4

350 g/12 oz wholewheat spaghetti

30 ml/2 tbsp olive oil

2 onions, finely chopped

225 g/8 oz lean minced (ground) pork

150 ml/¼ pt/⅔ cup chicken or pork stock, made with ½ stock cube

15 ml/1 tbsp chopped fresh sage

30 ml/2 tbsp chopped fresh parsley

12 cherry tomatoes, halved

200 ml/7 fl oz/scant 1 cup low-fat crème fraîche

Salt and freshly ground black pepper

50 g/2 oz/½ cup grated low-fat Mozzarella cheese

25 g/1 oz/¼ cup freshly grated Parmesan cheese, plus extra for dusting

To serve:

A green salad

---

1 Cook the spaghetti according to the packet directions. Drain and return to the pan.

2 Meanwhile, heat the oil in a separate saucepan, add the onions and pork and cook, stirring, for 5 minutes until the pork is no longer pink and all the grains are separate.

3 Add the stock and herbs, cover and simmer for 5 minutes. Add the tomatoes and cook for 2 minutes until they are just hot through but still holding their shape.

4 Stir in the crème fraîche and season to taste.

5 Tip the mixture into the pan of spaghetti and toss gently until well mixed. Add the Mozzarella and Parmesan and toss again.

6 Pile on to warm plates and sprinkle with a little extra Parmesan.

7 Serve with a green salad.

Spring Rolls
with Prawn and Egg Rice

*Spring rolls are usually deep-fried and oozing with grease.
Here they are baked to melting, golden crispness and taste
fantastic! And without all that added fat, you'll find yourself
full but not fatigued.*

SERVES 4

For the spring rolls:

175 g/6 oz pork fillet, cut into very thin strips

15 ml/1 tbsp cornflour (cornstarch)

30 ml/2 tbsp sunflower oil

1 garlic clove, crushed

½ bunch of spring onions (scallions), finely chopped

4 mushrooms, thinly sliced

100 g/4 oz/2 cups beansprouts

50 g/2 oz/½ cup frozen peas, thawed

1.5 ml/¼ tsp ground ginger

45 ml/3 tbsp light soy sauce

4 sheets of filo pastry (paste)

For the rice:

225 g/8 oz/1 cup brown basmati rice

½ bunch of spring onions, cut into short lengths

50 g/2 oz/½ cup frozen peas

*100 g/4 oz cooked peeled prawns (shrimp),
thawed if frozen*

2.5 ml/½ tsp Chinese five-spice powder

1 egg, beaten

1 Mix the pork with the cornflour.

2 Heat 15 ml/1 tbsp of the oil in a frying pan (skillet) over a high heat and fry (sauté) the pork for 1 minute, stirring. Add all the remaining spring roll ingredients except for 15 ml/1 tbsp of the soy sauce and the pastry, and stir-fry for 3 minutes. Remove from the heat and leave to cool.

3 Preheat the oven to 190°C/375°F/gas 5/fan oven 170°C.

4 Lay the pastry sheets on a work surface and fold each one in half. Divide the pork mixture into four portions and spoon one on to the centre of one edge of each sheet. Fold in the sides, then roll up.

5 Place the rolls on a non-stick baking (cookie) sheet. Brush with the remaining oil. Bake in the oven for about 20 minutes until golden brown.

6 Meanwhile, cook the rice in plenty of boiling, lightly salted water in a large non-stick saucepan for 30 minutes, adding the onions and peas for the last 5 minutes' cooking. Drain thoroughly and return to the saucepan.

7 Add the prawns, five-spice powder and the remaining soy sauce and toss over a gentle heat until hot through. Push the rice to one side of the pan. Tilt the pan and tip in the beaten egg. Cook, gradually scrambling the egg and mixing it into the rice until all the egg is cooked and stirred in.

8 Pile on to warm plates with the pancake rolls and serve.

POULTRY MAIN MEALS

Chicken and turkey are low in saturated fat – especially if you don't eat the skin. Use them for quick, tasty meals for any occasion. They lend themselves particularly well to stir-frying – a great way of cooking that uses only the minimum of added fat.

Chicken and Oriental Vegetable Stir-fry with Soba Noodles

Soba noodles are delicious buckwheat noodles from Japan, which you can now buy in major supermarkets as well as ethnic food stores. You can use ordinary Chinese egg noodles if you prefer. This quick-cook meal will sustain you for hours.

SERVES 4

---

1 onion, halved and cut into chunky pieces

15 ml/1 tbsp sunflower oil

2 skinless chicken breasts, cut into strips

3 heads of pak choi, shredded

2 garlic cloves, finely chopped

1 × 225 g/8 oz/small can of water chestnuts, drained and sliced

1 × 225 g/8 oz/small can of bamboo shoots, drained

2.5 ml/½ tsp Chinese five-spice powder

60 ml/4 tbsp light soy sauce

30 ml/2 tbsp water

225 g/8 oz soba noodles

1 Separate the onion pieces into layers.

2 Heat the oil in a large wok or frying pan (skillet). Add the onion and stir-fry for 2 minutes. Add the chicken and stir-fry for 3 minutes.

3 Add the pak choi, garlic, water chestnuts, bamboo shoots and five-spice powder. Stir-fry for a further 2–3 minutes until cooked to your liking. Stir in 45 ml/ 3 tbsp of the soy sauce and all the water.

4 Meanwhile, cook the noodles according to the packet directions. Drain well and toss with the remaining 15 ml/1 tbsp soy sauce.

5 Divide the noodles between four large warm bowls or plates. Spoon the chicken mixture over.

6 Serve straight away.

Swiss Cheese, Chicken and Fennel Salad

This crunchy salad contains a fabulous mixture of flavours and textures to tickle the taste buds. It is carefully balanced to sustain you without giving you that bloated feeling that brings on the yawns!

SERVES 4

4 skinless chicken breasts

45 ml/3 tbsp sunflower or olive oil

5 ml/1 tsp dried tarragon

Salt and freshly ground black pepper

100 g/4 oz/1 cup pine nuts

1 fennel bulb, sliced, reserving the green fronds for garnishing

100 g/4 oz/1 cup cubed Emmental (Swiss) cheese

1 red eating (dessert) apple, diced

100 g/4 oz green seedless grapes, halved

45 ml/3 tbsp low-fat crème fraîche

45 ml/3 tbsp low-fat mayonnaise

15 ml/1 tbsp lemon juice

5 ml/1 tsp clear honey

30 ml/2 tbsp chopped fresh parsley

4 large outer iceberg lettuce leaves

1 Brush the chicken breasts with 15 ml/1 tbsp of the oil, sprinkle with the tarragon and season lightly. Heat a griddle pan and cook the chicken for about 5 minutes on each side until cooked through and marked with dark griddle stripes on each side. Alternatively, you can grill (broil) the chicken.

2 Meanwhile, dry-fry the pine nuts in a frying pan (skillet) for a few minutes, tossing until lightly toasted. Remove from the pan straight away and reserve.

3 Mix the fennel with the cheese, apple and grapes. Blend the crème fraîche, mayonnaise and lemon juice together with the honey and season to taste with salt and pepper. Add to the cheese mixture and toss gently, adding half the parsley.

4 Sit a lettuce leaf on each of four plates. Spoon the fennel mixture into each cupped leaf. Cut the chicken breasts diagonally into thick slices and arrange attractively on top.

5 Sprinkle with the remaining parsley and serve.

Warm Sesame Chicken Salad

A warm oriental-style salad packed with B- and C-vitamins, this colourful, delicious dish is easy to make. It is designed to give you all the goodness you need for the rest of the day without making you over-full.

SERVES 4

90 ml/6 tbsp pure orange juice

90 ml/6 tbsp pure apple juice

30 ml/2 tbsp lemon juice

60 ml/4 tbsp cider vinegar

60 ml/4 tbsp light soy sauce

10 ml/2 tsp clear honey

1 garlic clove, crushed

1.5 ml/¼ tsp Chinese five-spice powder

5 ml/1 tsp grated fresh root ginger

4 skinless chicken breasts

100 g/4 oz baby sweetcorn (corn) cobs,
cut into short lengths

100 g/4 oz thin French (green) beans,
cut into short lengths

15 ml/1 tbsp sesame seeds

15 ml/1 tbsp sesame oil

1 small head of Chinese leaves (stem lettuce), shredded

1 bunch of spring onions (scallions),
cut into short lengths

1 carrot, thinly pared with a potato peeler

5 cm/2 in piece of cucumber, thinly pared
with a potato peeler

100 g/4 oz/2 cups beansprouts

1 Put the juices, vinegar, soy sauce and honey in a large, shallow container. Add the garlic, five-spice powder and ginger and mix well.

2 Make several slashes in each chicken breast and place in the marinade. Turn over to coat completely, cover and leave in a cool place for at least 4 hours (or overnight) to marinate.

3 Cook the sweetcorn and beans in boiling water for 3 minutes. Drain, rinse with cold water and drain again.

4 Heat a large frying pan (skillet) or wok. Add the sesame seeds and toss quickly until golden. Tip out of the pan straight away so they don't burn.

5 Heat the oil in the same pan. Cook the chicken breasts for about 6 minutes on each side until tender and cooked through. Add the marinade and simmer for 1 minute. Remove from the heat and leave to cool slightly.

6 Mix the cooked sweetcorn and beans with the Chinese leaves, spring onions, carrot, cucumber and beansprouts. Pile on four plates. Thickly slice the chicken breasts and arrange on top.

7 Spoon the warm marinade over and sprinkle with the toasted sesame seeds before serving.

Tandoori Chicken Breasts with Dhal

Low in fat and high in energy-giving nutrients, this dish is one of my favourites. The dhal also makes a good accompaniment for chops or steaks that have been spread with a little curry paste before grilling.

SERVES 4

4 skinless chicken breasts

For the marinade:

300 ml/¹/₂ pt/1¹/₄ cups plain low-fat yoghurt

1 small garlic clove, crushed

15 ml/1 tbsp tandoori powder

5 ml/1 tsp chopped fresh coriander (cilantro)

Salt and freshly ground black pepper

For the dhal:

175 g/6 oz/1 cup red lentils

1 onion, chopped

1 large garlic clove, crushed

15 ml/1 tbsp ground turmeric

15 ml/1 tbsp ground cumin

15 ml/1 tbsp ground coriander

10 ml/2 tsp paprika

600 ml/1 pt/2¹/₂ cups vegetable stock, made with 1 stock cube

Shredded lettuce, wedges of lemon and tomato and sprigs of coriander, for garnishing

1 Make several slashes in the flesh of the chicken. Mix together the remaining ingredients for the marinade in a large, shallow dish. Add the chicken and turn, pressing the mixture well into the slits. When well coated, leave to marinate for at least 3 hours.

2 Preheat the oven to 200°C/400°F/gas 6/fan oven 180°C. Place the chicken in a baking tin (pan). Spoon any remaining marinade over. Cover with foil. Bake in the oven for 20 minutes.

3 Remove the foil from the chicken and bake for a further 15 minutes or until browned in places and cooked through.

4 Meanwhile, put all the ingredients for the dhal in a saucepan and cook over a high heat until bubbling, stirring occasionally.

5 Skim off any scum from the surface with a draining spoon, then turn down the heat until gently bubbling round the edges.

6 Cook for 20–30 minutes until pulpy, stirring frequently to prevent the mixture sticking. If you think it is becoming too dry, add a little more water.

7 Spoon the dhal on to warm plates and put the chicken to one side.

8 Serve garnished with shredded lettuce, wedges of lemon and tomato and coriander leaves.

Baked Turkey Risotto with Mozzarella

So easy you could almost make it in your sleep! But this dish is packed with rice for energising slow-release carbohydrate, and turkey and cheese for protein and those all-important vitamins and minerals. With passata for vitamin C too, it's guaranteed to help you feel bright and ready for action.

SERVES 4

60 ml/4 tbsp olive oil

1 large onion, finely chopped

350 g/12 oz turkey stir-fry meat

350 g/12 oz/1½ cups risotto rice

900 ml/1½ pts/3¾ cups chicken stock, made with 2 stock cubes

Salt and freshly ground black pepper

1 bay leaf

30 ml/2 tbsp chopped fresh basil

75 g/3 oz/¾ cup grated low-fat Mozzarella cheese

For the tomato sauce:

300 ml/½ pt/1¼ cups passata (sieved tomatoes)

1 garlic clove, crushed

5 ml/1 tsp clear honey

To serve:

Freshly grated Parmesan cheese and a green salad

---

1 Preheat the oven to 180°C/350°F/gas 4/fan oven 160°C. Heat 60 ml/4 tbsp of the oil in a flameproof casserole (Dutch oven).

2 Add the onion and turkey and fry (sauté), stirring, for 2 minutes.

3   Stir in the rice until every grain is glistening with oil. Stir in the stock, add the bay leaf, season well and bring to the boil. Stir well again. Cover tightly and bake in the oven for 1 hour. Stir in half the basil, taste and re-season, if necessary. Sprinkle the Mozzarella over, cover and leave to stand to allow the cheese to melt.

4   Meanwhile, make the tomato sauce. Heat the passata, garlic, honey and a little salt and pepper in a small saucepan, stirring. Stir in the remaining basil.

5   Spoon the baked rice on to warm plates and trickle a little tomato sauce over.

6   Serve with grated Parmesan cheese and a green salad.

Turkey, Pineapple and Pepper Paella

Here's another great dish for any time of day and any occasion. It is made in one pan and as well as being quick and easy to prepare, provides you with all the health-giving nutrients you need. If you use white rice, cook it for 20–25 minutes only.

SERVES 4

---

15 ml/1 tbsp sunflower or olive oil

1 onion, chopped

1 garlic clove, crushed

350 g/12 oz diced turkey thigh meat

225 g/8 oz/1 cup brown basmati rice

2.5 ml/$^{1}/_{2}$ tsp ground cumin

1 × 225 g/8 oz/small can of pineapple pieces in natural juice, drained, reserving the juice

About 450 ml/$^{3}/_{4}$ pt/2 cups boiling water

1 chicken stock cube

100 g/4 oz whole baby button mushrooms

1 red (bell) pepper, diced

1 green pepper, diced

50 g/2 oz/$^{1}/_{2}$ cup frozen peas

2.5 ml/$^{1}/_{2}$ tsp dried oregano

Freshly ground black pepper

30 ml/2 tbsp chopped fresh parsley

---

1 Heat the oil in a large, heavy-based shallow pan. Add the onion, garlic and turkey and fry (sauté), stirring, for 3 minutes. Add the rice and cumin and stir until the grains are coated and glistening.

2 Add the pineapple pieces. Make the pineapple juice up to 600 ml/1 pt/2½ cups with the boiling water. Crumble in the stock cube. Stir, then add to the pan and bring to the boil, stirring all the time.

3 Add all the remaining ingredients except the parsley. Cover tightly, reduce the heat to as low as possible and cook very gently for 50 minutes. Stir and check everything is tender and the liquid has been absorbed. The rice should be moist and creamy, like a risotto. If not, re-cover and cook for a few more minutes.

4 Serve on warm plates, garnished with chopped parsley.

Thai-style Turkey with Sesame Seeds

This is yet another tasty, really easy dish that will give you all of the energy-boosting goodness you need. It can be made with chicken or pork, too, for a change.

SERVES 4

350 g/12 oz turkey stir-fry meat

1 red onion, halved and thinly sliced

1 red chilli, seeded and chopped

Finely grated zest and juice of 1 lime

Finely grated zest and juice of ½ lemon

1 garlic clove, crushed

15 ml/1 tbsp Thai fish sauce

5 ml/1 tsp clear honey

5 ml/1 tsp crushed lemon grass

5 ml/1 tsp sesame oil

15 ml/1 tbsp sunflower oil

30 ml/2 tbsp sesame seeds

Salt and freshly ground black pepper

225 g/8 oz rice noodles

1 red (bell) pepper, cut into very fine strips

1 green pepper, cut into very fine strips

30 ml/2 tbsp light soy sauce

½ small head of Chinese leaves (stem lettuce), shredded

30 ml/2 tbsp balsamic vinegar

1 Put the turkey and onion in a bowl. Add the chilli, the zest and juice of the lime and lemon, the garlic, fish sauce, honey, lemon grass, sesame and sunflower oils, sesame seeds and a little salt and pepper. Stir well and leave to marinate for 2 hours.

2 Cook the rice noodles according to the packet directions. Drain.

3 Cook the strips of pepper in boiling water for 4 minutes. Drain and keep warm.

4 Heat a large wok or frying pan (skillet). Add the turkey mixture and stir-fry for 4–5 minutes until cooked through. Stir in half of the soy sauce.

5 Put the shredded Chinese leaves in a salad bowl with the balsamic vinegar and the remaining soy sauce. Toss with a little black pepper.

6 Spoon the noodles into warm bowls. Top with the turkey mixture and then the mixed pepper strips. Serve straight away with the dressed Chinese leaves.

Chicken and Ginger Stir-fry

The brown rice will give you lots of sustained energy, and the multitude of fresh vegetables and chicken provide vital nutrients to keep you alert. Finally, there's a dash of fresh ginger, which is great for brain power.

SERVES 4

175 g/6 oz/³⁄₄ cup brown basmati rice

30 ml/2 tbsp sunflower oil

225 g/8 oz chicken stir-fry meat

5 ml/1 tsp grated fresh root ginger

1 bunch of spring onions (scallions), cut into short lengths

1 red (bell) pepper, cut into thin strips

1 carrot, cut into thin matchsticks

¼ cucumber, cut into matchsticks

¼ small green cabbage, cut into thin shreds

100 g/4 oz button mushrooms, sliced

100 g/4 oz/2 cups beansprouts

150 ml/¼ pt/²⁄₃ cup chicken stock, made with ½ stock cube

15 ml/1 tbsp light soy sauce

1 Cook the rice in plenty of boiling, lightly salted water for 30 minutes or according to the packet directions. Drain.

2 Meanwhile, heat the oil in a large frying pan (skillet) or wok. Add the chicken, ginger, onions, pepper and carrot and stir-fry for 4 minutes.

3 Add the cucumber, cabbage, mushrooms and beansprouts and stir-fry for a further 2 minutes. Add the stock and soy sauce and bring to the boil. Reduce the heat, cover with a lid and cook for 2 minutes.

4 Spoon the rice into bowls.

5 Pile the chicken stir-fry on top and serve.

FISH MAIN MEALS

Fish is a vital part of your fatigue-fighting regime. It contains essential oils, vitamins and minerals to keep you alert as well as being low in saturated fat and high in protein. Enjoy eating the many different varieties of seafood at least twice a week. This chapter contains plenty of ideas for delicious ways to cook them, all served with complex carbohydrates to help keep up your energy levels.

Brittany-style Mussels with Carrot and Celery

Using cider won't ruin your new high-energy diet because, once it's been boiled, the alcohol level is reduced to nothing. However, I have suggested apple juice as an alternative, if you prefer.

SERVES 4

1.75 kg/4 lb mussels, in their shells

40 g/1½ oz/3 tbsp low-fat sunflower, soya or olive oil spread

1 large onion, finely chopped

1 celery stick, finely chopped

1 large carrot, finely chopped

200 ml/7 fl oz/scant 1 cup cider or pure apple juice

120 ml/4 fl oz/½ cup water

Freshly ground black pepper

30 ml/2 tbsp chopped fresh parsley

To serve:

Rustic French bread and a large mixed salad

1 Scrub the mussels and scrape off any barnacles with a knife.

2 Discard any that are broken and any that are open and won't close when sharply tapped with the knife.

3 Pull off the 'beards' (the threads hanging down from the shells).

4 Melt the low-fat spread in a large saucepan and add the onion, celery and carrot. Cover and cook over a gentle heat for 3 minutes until softened but not browned.

5 Add the mussels, cider or apple juice and water and a good grinding of pepper.

6 Bring to the boil, cover and cook for about 5 minutes, shaking the pan occasionally until the mussels open. Discard any that remain closed.

7 Spoon the mussels into large, warm bowls with their cooking juices and sprinkle with parsley. Serve with rustic French bread to mop up the juices, followed by a large mixed salad.

Steamed Salmon in Lettuce with Pimiento and Chopped Egg Vinaigrette

I like to use large spinach leaves for this (blanch them in boiling water for 30 seconds before wrapping up the fish). But these days they are very hard to come by, unless you grow your own, so I use round lettuce leaves instead. Cook the potatoes in the simmering steaming water.

SERVES 4

For the vinaigrette:

2 eggs

60 ml/4 tbsp olive oil

30 ml/2 tbsp sunflower oil

30 ml/2 tbsp white wine vinegar

5 ml/1 tsp clear honey

10 ml/2 tsp Dijon mustard

Salt and freshly ground black pepper

30 ml/2 tbsp chopped fresh parsley

30 ml/2 tbsp snipped fresh chives

For the fish:

8–12 large round lettuce leaves

1 × 200 g/7 oz/small can of pimiento caps, drained and chopped

4 pieces of thick salmon fillet, 150 g/5 oz each, skinned

Chive stalks or sprigs of parsley, for garnishing

To serve:

New potatoes in their skins

1 Hard-boil (hard-cook) the eggs in boiling water for 7 minutes. Drain and plunge immediately into cold water. When cool enough to handle, peel and chop finely.

2 Whisk the oils, vinegar, honey and mustard together with a pinch of salt and a good grinding of pepper until thickened. Stir in the herbs and chopped egg and chill until ready to serve.

3 Cut any thick central stalks off the lettuce leaves. Take two or three of them (depending on size) and arrange overlapping on a board. Top with a quarter of the chopped pimiento, then a skinned salmon fillet. Season very lightly with salt and add a good grinding of pepper. Wrap the salmon in the leaves and place in a steamer or metal colander. Repeat with the remaining ingredients to make four parcels in all and pack them tightly side by side with the loosest edges underneath. Don't worry if they don't look too neat: once cooked, the lettuce will 'stick' to the fish.

4 Cover the steamer or colander with a lid and steam over a pan of simmering water for 10 minutes until the parcels feel firm.

5 Cut the parcels in half so you can see the fish and pimiento. Put two on each of four warm plates, resting one half on the other, so they look roughly stacked. Spoon a little dressing over, lay a few chive stalks or a sprig of parsley to one side of each to garnish.

6 Serve with new potatoes.

Grilled Mackerel with Mustard Seed and Raisin Couscous

Mackerel is a vastly underrated fish that is ideal on a fatigue-fighting diet. Here it is simply grilled, then served on a bed of high-energy couscous, flavoured with sweet raisins and mustard seeds for added nuttiness. The avocado in the salad provides phosphorus as well as other valuable vitamins and minerals.

SERVES 4

---

225 g/8 oz/1⅓ cups couscous

600 ml/1 pt/2½ cups boiling chicken or fish stock, made with 1 stock cube

4 mackerel, cleaned

Salt and freshly ground black pepper

15 ml/1 tbsp olive oil

30 ml/2 tbsp black mustard seeds

75 g/3 oz/½ cup raisins

10 ml/2 tsp lemon juice

30 ml/2 tbsp chopped fresh parsley

Wedges of lemon, for garnishing

To serve:

A green salad, including sliced avocado

---

1 Put the couscous in a bowl and add the boiling stock. Stir well. Sit the bowl over a pan of gently simmering water and steam for 10–20 minutes until tender.

2 Preheat the grill (broiler). Remove the heads from the mackerel, if you prefer, and make several slashes on each side of the flesh. Season the fish with just a sprinkling of salt and lots of black pepper.

3 Lay the fish on foil on the grill rack and grill (broil) for about 5 minutes on each side until golden and cooked through.

4 Heat the oil in a frying pan (skillet). Add the mustard seeds and heat until they begin to pop. Remove from the heat and stir in the raisins, lemon juice and parsley.

5 Add this mixture to the couscous and stir well with a fork to mix.

6 Spoon the couscous on to four warm plates. Set a mackerel on each and garnish with wedges of lemon.

7 Serve with a green salad including avocado.

Smoked Salmon, Potato and Broccoli Bake

Another perfect combination of textures and flavours, packed with all the nutrients you need. This also makes a fabulous starter for 8–12 people, served in small portions with a trickle of the sauce spooned over.

SERVES 4–6

3 large potatoes, scrubbed and diced

225 g/8 oz broccoli, cut into small florets

A little low-fat sunflower, soya or olive oil spread, for greasing

175 g/6 oz smoked salmon trimmings

3 large eggs

600 ml/1 pt/2½ cups milk

30 ml/2 tbsp freshly grated Parmesan cheese

Salt and freshly ground black pepper

15 ml/1 tbsp fresh chopped dill (dill weed)

For the sauce:

150 ml/¼ pt/⅔ cup low-fat crème fraîche

60 ml/4 tbsp milk

15 ml/1 tbsp chopped fresh dill

15 ml/1 tbsp snipped fresh chives

Finely grated zest and juice of ½ lemon

5 ml/1 tsp clear honey

Wedges of lemon and sprigs of dill, for garnishing

To serve:

A crisp green salad

1 Preheat the oven to 190°C/375°F/gas 5/fan oven 170°C.

2 Cook the potatoes in boiling, lightly salted water for about 4 minutes, then add the broccoli and cook for another 4 minutes, until both vegetables are just tender. Drain.

3 Grease a fairly large rectangular ovenproof serving dish (I use my lasagne dish). Tip in the potatoes and broccoli.

4 Break up the smoked salmon trimmings and scatter them over the vegetables. Turn over gently with a spoon to distribute evenly.

5 Beat the eggs and milk together with the Parmesan and season with a tiny pinch of salt and lots of pepper. Pour over the salmon mixture. Sprinkle with the dill.

6 Bake in the oven for about 45 minutes until golden and set.

7 Meanwhile, make the sauce. Whisk the crème fraîche and milk together until smooth, then stir in the remaining ingredients and season to taste. Chill until ready to serve.

8 Cut the warm bake into portions and place on plates, with a little of the cold sauce spooned over a corner of each one. Garnish each plate with a wedge of lemon and a sprig of fresh dill.

9 Serve with a crisp green salad.

Spiced Fresh Tuna with Crushed Chick Peas

The fragrant chick peas make a flavoursome, fatigue-busting accompaniment for tender, succulent fresh tuna. This dish has the added bonus of vitamin-C-rich tomatoes and, when served with an avocado and cucumber salad, is enriched with other vital vitamins and minerals.

SERVES 4

45 ml/3 tbsp olive or sunflower oil

10 ml/2 tsp ground cumin

5 ml/1 tsp coarsely crushed black peppercorns

Salt

4 fillets of fresh tuna, about 150 g/5 oz each

1 onion, finely chopped

1 garlic clove, crushed

2 × 425 g/15 oz/large cans of chick peas (garbanzos), drained

30 ml/2 tbsp chopped fresh coriander (cilantro)

3 tomatoes, skinned and diced

A squeeze of lemon juice

A few coriander leaves, for garnishing

To serve:

An avocado and cucumber salad

1 Mix 30 ml/2 tbsp of the oil with the cumin, pepper and a pinch of salt and rub over both sides of the tuna.

2 Heat the remaining oil in a saucepan. Add the onion and garlic and fry (sauté), stirring, for 3 minutes until lightly golden. Tip the chick peas into the pan and crush with a fork or the back of a wooden spoon against the sides of the pan, before stirring into the onion and garlic.

3 Stir in the coriander, tomatoes and lemon juice and heat through over a very low heat.

4 Meanwhile, preheat the grill (broiler). Place the tuna on foil on the grill rack and grill (broil) for 3–4 minutes on each side until just cooked but still slightly pink in the centre.

5 Pile the crushed chick pea mixture on to warm plates and top each with a tuna steak. Garnish with a few coriander leaves.

6 Serve with an avocado and cucumber salad.

Tomato Risotto
with Pesto Lemon Sole

*Here the risotto is cooked in vitamin-C-packed tomato juice
and the fish is wrapped round a filling high in B-complex
vitamins. The sole has fatigue-fighting minerals and the rice
gives you the all-important complex carbohydrates.
Serve with a rocket salad.*

SERVES 4

For the risotto:

15 ml/1 tbsp olive oil

1 onion, finely chopped

225 g/8 oz/1 cup risotto rice

*300 ml/^{1}/$_2$ pt/1^1/$_4$ cups boiling vegetable stock,
made with 1 stock cube*

450 ml/^{3}/$_4$ pt/2 cups tomato juice

*4 large lemon sole fillets, about 175 g/6 oz each,
skinned*

30 ml/2 tbsp pesto

100 g/4 oz/^{1}/$_2$ cup low-fat soft cheese

Salt and freshly ground black pepper

2.5 ml/^{1}/$_2$ tsp clear honey

To serve:

A rocket salad

1 Heat the oil in a saucepan. Add the onion and cook, stirring, over a gentle heat for 2 minutes until softened but not browned.

2 Add the rice and stir for 30 seconds until each grain of rice is coated in oil and glistening.

3 Add half the stock (reserve the rest for cooking the fish), bring back to the boil, turn down the heat and cook gently, stirring occasionally, until it is absorbed.

4   Add a third of the tomato juice, bring to the boil, turn down the heat again and cook, stirring occasionally, until the juice is absorbed. Repeat with the remaining tomato juice, adding half at a time until the juice is absorbed and the rice is creamy but still with some bite.

5   Meanwhile, lay the fish, skinned sides up, on a board. Spread with the pesto, then the soft cheese. Roll up and place in a frying pan (skillet). Pour the reserved stock around. Bring to the boil. Turn down the heat until gently bubbling around the edges. Cover with foil or a lid and cook for about 4–5 minutes until cooked through.

6   Season the risotto to taste with salt, pepper and the honey – it should be creamy but the rice should still have some 'bite'. If necessary, add a tablespoon or two of boiling water.

7   Spoon the risotto on to warm plates. Top with the fish and spoon the pan juices over.

Smoked Oyster and Tuna Rice Cakes on Vegetable Stir-fry

This dish has all the ingredients you need to fight tiredness. Oysters, whether fresh or smoked, are rich in zinc and phosphorus, as is tuna. Mixed with a medley of nutrient-rich vegetables and slow-release-energy rice, they make another winning recipe!

SERVES 4

100 g/4 oz/¹/₂ cup risotto rice

1 × 85 g/3¹/₂ oz/small can of smoked oysters, drained

1 × 85 g/3¹/₂ oz/very small can of tuna, drained

2 spring onions (scallions), chopped

30 ml/2 tbsp light soy sauce

A good pinch of Chinese five-spice powder

Freshly ground black pepper

1 egg, beaten

45 ml/3 tbsp sunflower oil

1 × 250 g/9 oz packet of fresh stir-fry vegetables with beansprouts

5 ml/1 tsp grated fresh root ginger

5 ml/1 tsp clear honey

1 Cook the rice in plenty of boiling, lightly salted water for about 20 minutes or until really tender. Drain, rinse with cold water and drain again.

2 Mash the oysters and tuna in a bowl with a fork. Add the cooked rice and the spring onions and mix well.

3 Add 15 ml/1 tbsp of the soy sauce, the five-spice powder, some pepper and the egg to the fish mixture and mix thoroughly.

4 Heat 30 ml/2 tbsp of the sunflower oil in a large, non-stick frying pan (skillet). Shape the mixture into eight small cakes. Fry (sauté) for 2–3 minutes until golden underneath. Turn them over and brown the other sides for a further 2–3 minutes. Drain on kitchen paper (paper towels) and keep warm.

5 Meanwhile, heat the remaining oil in a separate frying pan or wok. Add the packet of vegetables and stir-fry for 3 minutes. Stir in the ginger, honey and remaining 15 ml/1 tbsp soy sauce. Toss well.

6 Pile the stir-fry on warm plates and top with the fish cakes.

Braised Cod Loin on Puy Lentils

Cod loin is meaty and succulent. You could use monkfish or huss if you prefer. Whichever fish you use, when cooked with fragrant lentils and crisp vegetables it creates a wonderful, vibrant dish to fill you with vitality.

SERVES 4

30 ml/2 tbsp olive oil

4 pieces of cod loin, about 100 g/4 oz each

1 large red onion, chopped

1 celery stick, chopped

1 carrot, chopped

1 large garlic clove, crushed

450 ml/³/₄ pt/2 cups passata (sieved tomatoes)

15 ml/1 tbsp tomato purée (paste)

300 ml/¹/₂ pt/1¹/₄ cups dry white wine or grape juice

225 g/8 oz/1¹/₃ cups Puy lentils, rinsed

1 bay leaf

2 courgettes (zucchini), chopped

5 ml/1 tsp clear honey

Salt and freshly ground black pepper

15 ml/1 tbsp chopped fresh parsley, for garnishing

To serve:

Wholegrain bread and a green salad

1 Heat the oil in a flameproof casserole (Dutch oven) and brown the fish quickly on both sides. Remove from the pan.

2 Add the onion, celery, carrot and garlic and fry (sauté), stirring, for 2 minutes.

3 Add the passata, tomato purée, wine or juice and lentils. Stir and add the bay leaf. Bring to the boil, reduce the heat, cover and simmer gently for 45 minutes.

4 Stir in the courgettes and honey and season with a little salt and lots of pepper.

5 Lay the fish on top. Cover and continue to simmer for 15 minutes until the fish and lentils are tender. Discard the bay leaf.

6 Spoon the fish and lentils on to warm plates and sprinkle with parsley.

7 Serve with wholegrain bread and a green salad.

Low-fat Fish and Chips

So now you can enjoy Britain's favourite meal with all the flavour but none of the doziness that would ensue after a visit to the chippy! Note that oven chips are not suitable – they contain too much fat.

SERVES 6

---

6 cod or haddock fillets, about 150 g/5 oz each, skinned

150 g/5 oz/2½ cups fresh wholemeal breadcrumbs

30 ml/2 tbsp chopped fresh parsley

15 ml/1 tbsp chopped fresh thyme

15 ml/1 tbsp dried onion granules

Salt and freshly ground black pepper

2 egg whites

15 ml/1 tbsp water

450 g/1 lb frozen chips (fries)

Wedges of lemon and sprigs of watercress, for garnishing

To serve:

Peas and baby carrots

1 Preheat the oven to 220°C/425°F/gas 7/fan oven 200°C. Wipe the fish and remove any remaining bones.

2 Mix the breadcrumbs with half the parsley, all the thyme and dried onion granules and some salt and pepper in a shallow dish.

3 Beat the egg whites with the water in a separate dish.

4 Dip the fish in the egg white, then coat in the breadcrumbs. Place on a non-stick baking (cookie) sheet. Spread out the chips on a separate baking sheet.

5 Place the chips on the top shelf and the fish just below and bake for 30 minutes until golden and cooked.

6 Transfer the fish and chips to warm plates. Garnish with wedges of lemon and sprigs of watercress.

7 Serve with peas and baby carrots.

Fish Braise with Vegetables

The fish and vegetables give you all the nutrients you need to keep fresh and alert. Choose undyed smoked fish – this has all the goodness without added e-numbers, some of which may cause side effects.

SERVES 4

25 g/1 oz/2 tbsp low-fat sunflower, soya or olive oil spread

1 onion, thinly sliced

1 large carrot, thinly sliced

2 large potatoes, scrubbed and diced

¼ small green cabbage, shredded

1 × 400 g/14 oz/large can of chopped tomatoes

300 ml/½ pt/1¼ cups fish or vegetable stock, made with 1 stock cube

1 bouquet garni sachet

175 g/6 oz any chunky white fish, skinned and cubed

175 g/6 oz undyed smoked cod or haddock, skinned and cubed

100 g/4 oz raw peeled prawns (shrimp)

100 g/4 oz/1 cup frozen peas

Salt and freshly ground black pepper

15 ml/1 tbsp chopped fresh parsley, for garnishing

1 Heat the low-fat spread in a large saucepan and fry (sauté) the vegetables, stirring, for 2 minutes.

2 Stir in the tomatoes and stock, then the bouquet garni. Bring to the boil, part-cover, reduce the heat and simmer gently for 15 minutes. Remove the bouquet garni, squeezing it against the side of the pan.

3 Add the fish, prawns and peas, bring back to the boil, turn down the heat, re-cover and simmer for a further 5 minutes or until the fish and vegetables are tender. Season to taste and stir gently.

4 Ladle into warm bowls, sprinkle with parsley and serve.

Caribbean Prawn and Pasta Salad

Here you have a great combination of prawns for phosphorus and zinc and pasta for slow-release energy. Enjoy it as a TV supper – or even as a packed lunch!

SERVES 4

175 g/6 oz conchiglie (pasta shells)

1 × 225 g/8 oz/small can of pineapple chunks in natural juice, drained, reserving the juice

45 ml/3 tbsp low-fat mayonnaise

Finely grated zest and juice of 1 lime

60 ml/4 tbsp sunflower oil

3 celery sticks, chopped

2 carrots, grated

50 g/2 oz/¹/₃ cup stoned (pitted) dates, chopped

225 g/8 oz cooked peeled prawns (shrimp)

Salt and freshly ground black pepper

Lettuce leaves

A few coriander (cilantro) leaves, torn

1   Cook the pasta according to the packet directions. Drain, rinse with cold water and drain again.

2   Whisk 45 ml/3 tbsp of the pineapple juice with the mayonnaise, the zest and juice of the lime and the oil.

3   Add the cooked pasta and all the remaining ingredients except the lettuce and coriander and toss lightly. Season to taste, if necessary.

4   Arrange the lettuce leaves in a large serving bowl and pile the pasta mixture on top. Scatter the coriander over.

Tuna Niçoise

This fabulous mixture of vegetables and fish makes a great revitalising meal. The flavours complement each other perfectly, in fact you could close your eyes and imagine you're somewhere in the Mediterranean … but I guarantee you wouldn't be tempted to fall asleep!

SERVES 4

---

225 g/8 oz French (green) beans, cut into short lengths

225 g/8 oz new potatoes, scrubbed and diced

100 g/4 oz/1 cup frozen peas

2 hard-boiled (hard-cooked) eggs, roughly cut up

1 small onion, sliced into rings

4 tomatoes, roughly diced

1 × 185 g/6½ oz/small can of tuna, drained

1 × 50 g/2 oz/small can of anchovies, drained and cut into thin slivers

90 ml/6 tbsp olive oil

30 ml/2 tbsp red wine vinegar

Salt and freshly ground black pepper

½ cos (romaine) lettuce, cut into bite-sized pieces

Whole lettuce leaves

A few black olives

---

1 Cook the beans, potatoes and peas for 5 minutes in boiling, lightly salted water until just tender. Drain, rinse with cold water and drain again.

2 Place in a bowl with all the remaining ingredients except the whole lettuce leaves and olives and season with lots of black pepper. Toss very gently so as not to break up the tuna.

3 Pile on to a bed of lettuce leaves and scatter a few black olives over.

Rustic Salmon
with Camargue Red Rice

*Camargue red rice has a wonderful nutty texture and flavour.
Brown basmati and even wild rice make equally delicious
alternatives (but cook these for 15 minutes before adding the
fish and beans). Whichever you choose, their distinctive
flavours and colours will complement the succulent salmon
and vegetables perfectly.*

SERVES 4

---

25 g/1 oz/2 tbsp low-fat sunflower, soya or olive oil spread

1 onion, chopped

1 leek, sliced

1 sweet potato, diced

1 carrot, diced

100 g/4 oz/¹/₂ cup Camargue red rice

1 × 400 g/14 oz/large can of chopped tomatoes

450 ml/³/₄ pt/2 cups fish stock, made with 1 stock cube

Salt and freshly ground black pepper

2.5 ml/¹/₂ tsp dried oregano

450 g/1 lb salmon fillet, skinned and cut into chunks

100 g/4 oz French (green) beans, cut into short lengths

1 Heat the low-fat spread in a large flameproof casserole (Dutch oven). Add the onion, leek, potato and carrot and fry (sauté), stirring, for 3 minutes.

2 Stir in the rice, then add the tomatoes, stock, a pinch of salt, some pepper and the oregano. Bring to the boil, stirring, then reduce the heat, cover and simmer gently for 10 minutes.

3 Add the salmon and beans, re-cover and simmer for about 10 minutes or until the rice, fish and vegetables are tender.

4 Serve in warm bowls.

Crunchy Sardines with Lime

Fresh sardines are one of my favourite fish. When buying, look for bright eyes and gills, and firm bodies; if they are soft and soggy, they are not fresh. Oily fish are brilliant for fatigue-fighting and laced with vitamin-C-rich limes, they are superb. Enjoy them with tabbouleh for slow-release energy or with rustic bread and salad.

SERVES 4–6

1 kg/2¼ lb fresh sardines, cleaned

Finely grated zest and juice of 1 lime

Freshly ground black pepper

50 g/2 oz/½ cup oat bran

50 g/2 oz/1 cup bran flakes, crushed

45 ml/3 tbsp sesame seeds

30 ml/2 tbsp olive or sunflower oil

Wedges of lime and sprigs of parsley, for garnishing

To serve:

Tabbouleh (see page 154)

1 Scrape any large scales off the sardines, then rinse well and pat dry on kitchen paper (paper towels).

2 Preheat the oven to 200°C/400°F/gas 6/fan oven 180°C. Lay the fish on a non-stick baking (cookie) sheet. Sprinkle with the zest and juice of the lime and season with pepper on both sides.

3 Mix the oat bran, crushed bran flakes and sesame seeds together. Brush the fish all over with oil and coat in the seed mixture.

4 Bake on a shelf near the top of the oven for about 10–15 minutes until golden and cooked through. Garnish with wedges of limes and sprigs of parsley.

5 Serve with tabbouleh.

Thai-style King Prawn Stir-fry

This colourful dish contains so many healthy ingredients –
pak choi for folate, mushrooms and prawns for phosporus
and zinc, rice for slow-release energy – the whole lot makes
for a superb meal packed with vitality.

SERVES 4

30 ml/2 tbsp sunflower oil

3 heads of pak choi, cut into chunks

100 g/4 oz button mushrooms, sliced

1 bunch of spring onions (scallions), cut into short lengths

1 large garlic clove, crushed

1 green chilli, seeded and finely chopped

30 ml/2 tbsp pickled sliced ginger

5 ml/1 tsp crushed lemon grass

450 g/1 lb raw peeled king prawns (jumbo shrimp),
tails left on, thawed if frozen

100 g/4 oz mangetout (snow peas)

Finely grated zest and juice of 1 lime

30 ml/2 tbsp Thai fish sauce

30 ml/2 tbsp chopped fresh coriander (cilantro)

To serve:

Thai fragrant rice

1 Heat the oil in a large frying pan (skillet) or wok. Add the pak choi, mushrooms and spring onions and stir-fry for 2 minutes.

2 Add the garlic, chilli, ginger and lemon grass and stir-fry for 30 seconds.

3 Add the prawns and mangetout and stir-fry for 2–3 minutes or until the prawns are pink.

4 Stir in the lime zest and juice, fish sauce and coriander and stir-fry for 1 minute.

5 Serve with Thai fragrant rice.

Steamed Trout with Asparagus on Chive Mash

Asparagus is rich in phosphorus and folate. Here it is served with fresh trout and mash, flavoured with chives, making a delicious meal, packed with vitality-inducing ingredients.

SERVES 4

For the mash:

4 large potatoes, cut into small pieces

1 onion, chopped

A knob of low-fat sunflower, soya or olive oil spread

30 ml/2 tbsp milk

30 ml/2 tbsp snipped fresh chives

Salt and freshly ground black pepper

225 g/8 oz thin short asparagus spears

4 rainbow trout fillets

2.5 ml/½ tsp finely grated lemon zest

2.5 ml/½ tsp herbes de Provence

Wedges of lemon, for garnishing

To serve:

Low-fat mayonnaise

1 Boil the potatoes and onion in very lightly salted water for about 10 minutes or until tender. Drain thoroughly, return to the pan and mash with the low-fat spread and milk. Beat in the chives and season to taste.

2 Meanwhile, line a steamer or metal colander with foil. Spread the asparagus out in a single layer on the foil. Lay the fish on top and sprinkle with the lemon zest, herbs and a very little salt and pepper. Cover and steam over a pan of boiling water for 10 minutes.

3 Pile the mash on warm plates and lay the fish and asparagus alongside. Garnish with wedges of lemon.

4 Serve with low-fat mayonnaise.

Honey-soused Mackerel

Mackerel is a great-tasting oily fish but if you find it a bit rich, you may like this treatment. Soused in vinegar and herbs, with a dash of honey to take away the acidity, it is lighter and full of subtle flavours.

SERVES 4

4 small mackerel, cleaned and boned

Salt and freshly ground black pepper

1 small onion, thinly sliced and separated into rings

15 ml/1 tbsp fresh chopped dill (dill weed), or 5 ml/1 tsp dried

300 ml/½ pt/1¼ cups white wine vinegar

300 ml/½ pt/1¼ cups water

15 ml/1 tbsp clear honey

1 large bay leaf

To serve:

New potatoes and a mixed salad

1 Preheat the oven to 180°C/350°F/gas 4/fan oven 160°C. Trim the fins and tails off the fish and open out flat.

2 Season the flesh very lightly with salt and add a good grinding of pepper.

3 Sprinkle with the onion rings and the dill. Roll up, skin-sides out, starting from the head ends. Place side by side in a shallow ovenproof dish.

4 Mix the vinegar with the water and honey and pour over. Tuck the bay leaf in between the fish.

5 Cover the dish with foil and bake in the oven for 45 minutes until cooked through. Leave to cool in the liquid.

6 Serve cold with new potatoes and a mixed salad.

VEGETARIAN MAIN MEALS

A vegetarian diet can be very good to fight fatigue, being high in starchy carbohydrates, but you must make sure you eat enough protein and vitamins. The recipes in this section have been specially chosen with this in mind. It is worth noting that the only vegetable source for vitamin B12 is found in yeast extract – so Marmite soldiers for breakfast are a great idea!

Green Tagliatelle with Leek, Gorgonzola and Walnut Sauce

A rich, creamy sauce, with heaps of flavour and packed with vitality-inducing ingredients. I use spinach-flavoured tagliatelle for this but wholewheat spaghetti is good too.

SERVES 4

350 g/12 oz green tagliatelle

50 g/2 oz/¼ cup low-fat sunflower, soya or olive oil spread

2 large leeks, thinly sliced

175 g/6 oz/1½ cups Gorgonzola, crumbled

120 ml/4 fl oz/½ cup low-fat crème fraîche

120 ml/4 fl oz/½ cup dry white wine or grape juice

50 g/2 oz/½ cup chopped walnuts

Salt and freshly ground black pepper

15 ml/1 tbsp lemon juice

A few flatleaf parsley leaves, torn, for garnishing

To serve:

A mixed salad

1 Cook the pasta according to the packet directions. Drain and return to the pan.

2 Meanwhile, melt the low-fat spread in a saucepan. Add the leeks and cook gently, stirring, for 2 minutes until softened.

3 Stir in the cheese until melted. Blend in the crème fraîche and wine or grape juice. Heat, stirring, until thickened – this should take about 1½ minutes. Stir in the nuts and season lightly.

4 Tip the sauce into the tagliatelle and toss to coat.

5 Spoon into bowls and scatter a few torn flatleaf parsley leaves over.

6 Serve with a mixed salad.

Cashew Nut Roast

This rich, revitalising dish is also good served with a vegetable gravy, baked potatoes and a green vegetable.

SERVES 4

---

150 g/5 oz/1¼ cups raw cashew nuts, chopped

75 g/3 oz/1½ cups fresh wholemeal breadcrumbs

1 red onion, finely chopped

15 ml/1 tbsp light soy sauce

2.5 ml/½ tsp dried oregano

5 ml/1 tsp lemon juice

25 g/1 oz/2 tbsp low-fat sunflower, soya or olive oil spread, plus a little for greasing

5 ml/1 tsp yeast extract

150 ml/¼ pt/⅔ cup hot water

For the sauce:

1 × 170 g/6 oz/small can of creamed mushrooms

A little milk

To serve:

Creamed potatoes, sweetcorn (corn) and Brussels sprouts

1 Preheat the oven to 190°C/375°F/gas 5/fan oven 170°C. Lightly grease a 1.2 litre/2 pt/5 cup ovenproof dish with a little low-fat spread.

2 Mix all the ingredients except the yeast extract and water.

3 Blend the yeast extract and water and stir into the mixture. Spoon everything into the prepared dish.

4 Bake in the oven for 30–40 minutes until golden brown and hot through.

5 Heat the mushrooms and thin to a pouring sauce with milk.

6 Slice the nut roast. Serve with the mushroom sauce, creamed potatoes, sweetcorn and Brussels sprouts.

Curried Soya Bean Roast with Spicy Dressing

Vegetarian nut and pulse roasts can be a bit dull but this loaf, with its spicy dressing, is packed full of flavour, as well as all the energy-giving properties you need in a meal. It is equally delicious served hot with a curry sauce and vegetables.

SERVES 6

2 × 425 g/15 oz/large cans of soya beans, drained

50 g/2 oz/¼ cup low-fat sunflower, soya or olive oil spread, plus a little for greasing

45 ml/3 tbsp dried breadcrumbs

1 large onion, finely chopped

1 carrot, grated

1 potato, grated

½ small swede (rutabaga), grated

15 ml/1 tbsp mild curry paste

50 g/2 oz/½ cup fresh wholemeal breadcrumbs

15 ml/1 tbsp clear honey

Salt and freshly ground black pepper

2 eggs, beaten

For the dressing:

90 ml/6 tbsp low-fat crème fraîche

45 ml/3 tbsp sunflower oil

5 ml/1 tsp garam masala

5 ml/1 tsp onion granules

5 ml/1 tsp lemon juice

30 ml/2 tbsp chopped fresh coriander (cilantro)

To serve:

A mixed salad

1 Tip the soya beans into a bowl and mash with a potato masher.

2 Grease a 900 g/2 lb loaf tin (pan) with a little low-fat spread and sprinkle with the dried breadcrumbs. Preheat the oven to 190°C/375°F/gas 5/fan oven 170°C.

3 Melt the measured low-fat spread in a saucepan over a moderate heat. Add the prepared vegetables and the curry paste and fry (sauté), stirring, for 5 minutes.

4 Stir this mixture into the soya beans with the fresh breadcrumbs and the honey. Season well.

5 Mix in the beaten eggs, then turn the mixture into the prepared tin and smooth the surface.

6 Cover the tin with foil and bake in the oven for 1½ hours until firm to the touch. Cool for 10 minutes in the tin, then turn out on to a serving dish.

7 Whisk the dressing ingredients together and season to taste.

8 Serve the loaf warm or cold, in slices, with the dressing spooned over, accompanied by a mixed salad.

Tomatoes Stuffed with Fragrant Brown Rice and Pistachios

This is a light but filling meal, packed with plenty of flavour and energy-boosting nutrients. Ring the changes with other nuts or seeds instead of the pistachios.

SERVES 4

8 beefsteak tomatoes

4 spring onions (scallions), finely chopped

25 g/1 oz/2 tbsp low-fat sunflower, soya or olive oil spread

100 g/4 oz/½ cup brown basmati rice

300 ml/½ pt/1¼ cups vegetable stock, made with 1 stock cube

Freshly ground black pepper

25 g/1 oz/¼ cup pistachio nuts, chopped

30 ml/2 tbsp currants

2 sprigs of fresh rosemary

Wedges of lemon, for garnishing

To serve:

A green salad and olive ciabatta bread

1 Cut a slice off each of the rounded ends of the tomatoes and reserve for 'lids'. Scoop out the seeds and reserve.

2 Fry (sauté) the onions in the low-fat spread for 2 minutes until softened but not browned.

3 Stir in the rice, stock and a little pepper (it should not require salt). Bring to the boil, reduce the heat, cover and simmer gently for 30 minutes.

4 Stir in the nuts, currants and rosemary and cook, uncovered, stirring occasionally, for a further 15 minutes or until the rice is really tender and has absorbed all the liquid.

5 Remove the rosemary, taste and re-season, if necessary. Stir in the tomato seeds, then pack the mixture into the tomatoes, replace the lids and chill.

6 Garnish with lemon wedges and serve with a green salad and olive ciabatta bread.

Aubergine, Potato and Lentil Madras

There is lots of slow-release energy in this. The salad is an important part of the meal as it creates the perfect balance.

SERVES 4

---

1 onion, sliced

30 ml/2 tbsp sunflower oil

1 garlic clove, crushed

2 large waxy potatoes, scrubbed and diced

1 large aubergine (eggplant), diced

15 ml/1 tbsp Madras curry paste

90 ml/6 tbsp water

150 ml/¼ pt/⅔ cup vegetable stock, made with ½ stock cube

2 × 425 g/15 oz/large cans of lentils, drained

100 g/4 oz/1 cup frozen peas

150 ml/¼ pt/⅔ cup plain low-fat yoghurt

30 ml/2 tbsp chopped fresh coriander (cilantro)

Salt and freshly ground black pepper

To serve:

Naan bread and a green salad

---

1   Fry (sauté) the onion in the oil for 2 minutes in a large saucepan. Add the garlic, potatoes, aubergine, curry paste and water and cook, stirring, for 2 minutes.

2   Add the stock, cover with a lid, reduce the heat and cook gently for 15 minutes.

3   Stir in the lentils, peas and yoghurt. Continue to cook gently, uncovered, for a further 15 minutes until everything is tender and bathed in sauce. Stir in the coriander and adjust the seasoning, if necessary.

4   Serve hot with naan bread and a green salad.

Mediterranean Vegetable Risotto with Basil

Polished risotto rice gives the best consistency, but you could use round-grain brown rice for added fibre.

SERVES 4

1 large onion, chopped

1 green (bell) pepper, diced

1 aubergine (eggplant), diced

1 courgette (zucchini), diced

45 ml/3 tbsp olive oil

225 g/8 oz/1 cup risotto rice

900 ml/1½ pts/3¾ cups vegetable stock, made with 2 stock cubes

1 × 400 g/14 oz/large can of chopped tomatoes

5 ml/1 tsp dried basil

Salt and freshly ground black pepper

30 ml/2 tbsp chopped fresh basil

100 g/4 oz/1 cup grated low-fat Mozzarella cheese

60 ml/4 tbsp freshly grated Parmesan cheese

To serve:

A rocket salad

1 Fry (sauté) all the prepared vegetables in the oil in a large saucepan for 5 minutes, stirring occasionally.

2 Add the rice and cook, stirring, for 1 minute.

3 Add all the remaining ingredients, except the basil and cheeses, and bring to the boil. Stir well, turn down the heat to as low as possible, cover with foil, then a lid, and cook for 20 minutes without stirring, until the rice is just tender and has absorbed all the liquid.

4 Stir in the basil and sprinkle with the grated Mozzarella and Parmesan.

5 Serve with a rocket salad.

Chick Pea and Vegetable Ragoût with Caraway

This is a form of goulash, which you can serve with noodles if you need added slow-release energy. Either way, it has lots of vitamins and minerals and plenty of flavour.

SERVES 4

30 ml/2 tbsp olive oil

1 onion, chopped

1 garlic clove, crushed

15 ml/1 tbsp paprika

2 large carrots, diced

1 celery stick, chopped

1 large potato, diced

100 g/4 oz button mushrooms, sliced

1 red (bell) pepper, diced

450 ml/³/₄ pt/2 cups vegetable stock, made with 1 stock cube

2.5 ml/¹/₂ tsp dried oregano

30 ml/2 tbsp tomato purée (paste)

15 ml/1 tbsp Worcestershire sauce

5 ml/1 tsp clear honey

15 ml/1 tbsp caraway seeds, plus extra for garnishing

Salt and freshly ground black pepper

2 × 425 g/15 oz/large cans of chick peas (garbanzos), drained

60 ml/4 tbsp low-fat crème fraîche, for garnishing

To serve:

A green salad

1 Heat the oil in a large saucepan. Add the onion and garlic and fry (sauté) for 2 minutes, stirring. Stir in the paprika and stir for 30 seconds.

2 Add all the remaining ingredients except the crème fraîche. Bring to the boil, turn down the heat, part-cover and simmer for 30 minutes or until all the vegetables are tender and bathed in a rich sauce. Taste and re-season, if necessary.

3 Ladle into warm bowls and top each with a spoonful of crème fraîche and a sprinkling of extra caraway seeds.

4 Serve with a green salad.

Spinach and Peanut Loaf with Leek and Tomato Sauce

Peanuts are a great source of zinc. In this recipe, they are combined with spinach (high in iron and folate) and a tomato sauce full of vitamin C.

SERVES 4

---

225 g/8 oz frozen spinach, thawed

1 large onion, quartered

1 garlic clove

175 g/6 oz/1½ cups raw peanuts

4 slices of wholemeal bread, torn into pieces

1 egg

5 ml/1 tsp yeast extract

5 ml/1 tsp dried thyme

Salt and freshly ground black pepper

A little sunflower oil, for greasing

2 large leeks, thinly sliced

15 g/½ oz/1 tbsp low-fat sunflower, soya or olive oil spread

150 ml/¼ pt/⅔ cup water

450 ml/¾ pt/2 cups passata (sieved tomatoes)

A good pinch of dried basil

To serve:

Jacket potatoes and French (green) beans

---

1 Preheat the oven to 180°C/350°F/gas 4/fan oven 160°C.

2 Squeeze out the spinach to remove as much moisture as possible. Place in a blender or food processor. Run the machine and drop in the onion, garlic, peanuts and bread. Blend until finely chopped but do not purée. Alternatively, pass the ingredients through a coarse mincer (grinder), adding the bread last.

3 Using a fork, briskly mix the egg with the yeast extract in a small bowl until well blended and stir into the spinach mixture with the thyme and a little salt and pepper.

4 Turn into a greased 450 g/1 lb loaf tin (pan) and cover with foil.

5 Bake in the oven for 1 hour or until firm to the touch.

6 Fry (sauté) the leeks in the low-fat spread for 2 minutes, stirring. Add the water and bring to the boil. Reduce the heat, cover and cook very gently for 10 minutes or until really tender. Remove the lid and boil rapidly to evaporate the water, stirring to prevent sticking.

7 Stir in the passata and basil and season to taste. Bring to the boil, reduce the heat and simmer for 3 minutes.

8 Leave the loaf to cool for 3–4 minutes, then turn out on to a warm serving dish.

9 Serve sliced, with the leek and tomato sauce, jacket potatoes and green beans.

Vegetable Satay
with Brown Rice and Beans

The peanuts in this sauce are rich in zinc, the vegetables and beans provide all your other 'energising' vitamins and minerals, and brown rice is for serious long-term energy.

SERVES 4

225 g/8 oz/1 cup brown basmati rice

1 × 425 g/15 oz/large can of borlotti beans, drained

2.5 ml/½ tsp ground cumin

1 small swede (rutabaga), cut into chunks

2 large carrots, cut into chunks

1 large parsnip, cut into chunks

2 courgettes (zucchini), cut into chunks

2 corn cobs, each cut into 4 pieces

15 g/½ oz/1 tbsp low-fat sunflower, soya or olive oil spread

15 ml/1 tbsp clear honey

150 ml/¼ pt/⅔ cup milk

75 ml/5 tbsp smooth peanut butter

1.5 ml/¼ tsp chilli powder

To serve:

Cucumber salad with yoghurt dressing

1   Soak eight wooden kebab skewers in cold water for 1 hour.

2   Cook the rice in plenty of boiling, lightly salted water for 30 minutes or until just tender. Drain, rinse with boiling water and drain again. Return to the pan and add the beans and cumin. Toss over a gentle heat until piping hot.

3 Meanwhile, put a large saucepan of lightly salted water over a high heat. When boiling, add the vegetables and cook for 4 minutes until almost tender. Drain.

4 When cool enough to handle, thread on the skewers. Lay them on foil on the grill (broiler) rack.

5 Melt the low-fat spread with the honey and brush all over the kebabs.

6 Cook under the grill (broiler) until golden, turning once or twice and brushing with more honey mixture.

7 Meanwhile, put the milk, peanut butter and chilli powder in a saucepan and heat gently, stirring, until the mixture forms a thick sauce.

8 Spoon the rice and beans on to four warm plates. Top with the kebabs and spoon the sauce over.

9 Serve with a cucumber salad with yoghurt dressing.

Potato and Tofu Sauté

Tofu is fermented bean curd, rich in vitamins, minerals and protein but low in fat. Here it is mixed with many health-giving ingredients to make an energy-boosting dish.

SERVES 4

---

700 g/1½ lb new potatoes, cut into bite-sized pieces

30 ml/2 tbsp pine nuts

25 g/1 oz/2 tbsp low-fat sunflower, soya or olive oil spread

1 bunch of spring onions (scallions), chopped

1 green (bell) pepper, diced

1 red pepper, diced

1 × 320 g/12 oz/medium can of sweetcorn (corn), drained

250 g/9 oz smoked tofu, cubed

15 ml/1 tbsp pimentón

5 ml/1 tsp dried thyme

Salt and freshly ground black pepper

30 ml/2 tbsp chopped fresh parsley

To serve:

A mixed salad

1 Boil the potatoes in water for 5 minutes. Drain.

2 Heat a large frying pan (skillet) or wok. Add the pine nuts and toss until golden, then remove from the pan immediately and set aside.

3 Melt the low-fat spread in the pan. Add the spring onions and peppers and fry (sauté) for 2 minutes, stirring.

4 Add the potatoes and continue to fry, stirring and turning, for 5 minutes until turning golden.

5 Add all the remaining ingredients except the pine nuts and parsley, season to taste with salt and pepper and continue to cook, stirring, for 3 minutes until everything is hot. Sprinkle with the pine nuts and parsley.

6 Serve straight from the pan with a mixed salad.

STIMULATING SIDE DISHES

All kinds of vegetables, whether fresh, canned (in water) or frozen, are good for you. The green and yellow varieties are particularly important for keeping you alert, the starchy ones are vital for slow-release energy and the skins that you eat give you vital fibre that stops you getting that sluggish feeling.

Boiled and steamed vegetables are quick and easy to prepare, but this section provides you with some innovative ways of serving them, together with tasty rice and pasta dishes that will liven up both you and your meal table.

Tabbouleh

Cracked wheat grains, mixed with herbs, garlic, olive oil and lemon juice, tabbouleh is a traditional North African dish that makes the perfect slow-release energy accompaniment to meat, fish or poultry as well as being a great snack meal on its own.

SERVES 4–6

225 g/8 oz/2 cups bulghar (cracked) wheat

4 spring onions (scallions), chopped

1 garlic clove, crushed

60 ml/4 tbsp chopped fresh parsley

30 ml/2 tbsp chopped fresh coriander (cilantro)

30 ml/2 tbsp chopped fresh mint

30 ml/2 tbsp lemon juice

60 ml/4 tbsp olive oil

Salt and freshly ground black pepper

¼ cucumber, finely chopped

4 ripe tomatoes, chopped

1 Put the bulghar in a large bowl. Cover with boiling water and leave to stand for 30 minutes. Stir with a fork to fluff up.

2 Add the spring onions, garlic, herbs, lemon juice and olive oil. Lift and stir until thoroughly mixed and leave until cold.

3 Stir in the cucumber and tomatoes. Chill until ready to serve.

Spicy Potato Wedges

No grease to sap your energy here – the potatoes are dipped in milk and spices, then baked until crisp and golden on the outside, soft in the middle. If you don't like spicy foods, simply dip the potato wedges in milk and sprinkle lightly with celery or garlic salt before baking.

SERVES 4

4 large potatoes, scrubbed

45 ml/3 tbsp milk

5 ml/1 tsp paprika

5 ml/1 tsp ground cumin

1.5 ml/¼ tsp chilli powder

5 ml/1 tsp garlic salt

Freshly ground black pepper

1 Preheat the oven to 200°C/400°F/gas 6/fan oven 180°C. Cut the potatoes into halves, then wedges.

2 Put the milk in a bowl. Add the potatoes and toss until well coated.

3 Mix the spices, garlic salt and a good grinding of pepper together.

4 Arrange the potato wedges on a non-stick baking (cookie) sheet. Sprinkle with half the spice mixture. Turn the wedges over and sprinkle the other sides.

5 Place on a shelf near the top of the oven and bake for about 25 minutes until crisp and deep golden brown (if you have cut them thinly, take care they don't burn). Turn over halfway through cooking.

6 Serve hot.

Hot Potato Salad

This is a great complex-carbohydrate accompaniment, which also makes a great snack meal on its own. The anchovies add phosphorus and A- and B-vitamins as well as lots of flavour!

SERVES 4–6

1 kg/2¼ lb medium potatoes, scrubbed

Salt

1 × 50 g/2 oz/small can of anchovies, drained

30 ml/2 tbsp milk

250 ml/8 fl oz/1 cup low-fat crème fraîche

5 ml/1 tsp lemon juice

Freshly ground black pepper

Paprika, for garnishing

1 Put the potatoes in a saucepan with enough cold water to cover. Add a good pinch of salt.

2 Cover and bring to the boil over a high heat, then cook for 10–15 minutes until really tender. Drain in a colander. When cool enough to handle, peel off the skins. Cut into chunks and return to the pan.

3 Meanwhile, soak the anchovies in milk for 5 minutes to remove excess salt. Drain. Reserve four anchovies for garnish and finely chop the remainder. Mix with the crème fraîche, lemon juice and a little pepper. Add to the potatoes and lift and stir lightly over a low heat.

4 Spoon into a warm serving dish. Cut the reserved anchovies into halves, lengthways. Arrange attractively on top and sprinkle with paprika.

5 Serve hot.

Mixed Vegetable Pilau Rice

This delicious, colourful accompaniment combines many of the vitamins, minerals and complex carbohydrates you need, in one dish. Enjoy it with any meat, poultry or fish – do not just save it for curries!

SERVES 4

Salt

5 ml/1 tsp ground turmeric

4–6 cardamom pods, split

2.5 cm/1 in piece of cinnamon stick

175 g/6 oz/³/₄ cup basmati rice

2 carrots, diced

1 green (bell) pepper, diced

1 courgette (zucchini), diced

¹/₂ small cauliflower, cut into tiny florets

15 ml/1 tbsp sunflower oil

1 onion, finely chopped

1 Bring a large pan of water to the boil and add a pinch of salt and the spices. Add the rice and carrots and boil for 6 minutes. Add the pepper, courgette and cauliflower and boil for a further 4 minutes until everything is tender. Drain in a colander.

2 Heat the oil in a frying pan (skillet) over a high heat and fry (sauté) the onion for 3–4 minutes until golden brown and soft.

3 Use a fork to mix the onion into the rice. Remove the spices, or not, as you wish.

4 Serve hot or cold.

Spinach and Lasagne Bake

This makes a perfect accompaniment to any simply-cooked meat, poultry or fish. I often serve it as a light meal with a home-made tomato sauce: lightly cook a chopped onion in just a trickle of olive oil, add a can of chopped tomatoes and simmer for a few minutes, then season with salt, pepper and a good pinch of dried basil. Easy!

SERVES 4

---

450 g/1 lb frozen chopped spinach, thawed and drained

1 garlic clove, crushed

2.5 ml/½ tsp dried oregano

200 g/7 oz/scant 2 cups low-fat soft cheese

Salt and freshly ground black pepper

30 ml/2 tbsp milk

6 sheets of no-need-to-precook lasagne

150 ml/¼ pt/⅔ cup low-fat crème fraîche

1 egg

60 ml/4 tbsp freshly grated Parmesan cheese

1 Preheat the oven to 190°C/375°F/gas 5/fan oven 170°C. Squeeze the spinach to remove most of the excess water. Mix with the garlic, oregano and soft cheese. Season lightly.

2 Put the milk in the base of a medium-sized, shallow, rectangular ovenproof dish.

3 Put two sheets of lasagne on top, breaking to fit, if necessary.

4 Spread half the spinach mixture on top, then top with two more sheets of lasagne, then the remaining spinach mixture, then the last two sheets of lasagne.

5 Beat the crème fraîche with the egg and Parmesan and season lightly. Spoon over the lasagne.

6 Bake in the oven for about 35 minutes until golden, set and cooked through. Serve cut into quarters.

Crispy Potato Skins

Greasy snacks will make you feel tired, so try these crunchy nibbles for a change. They're tasty and cheap too – the main ingredient is those potato peelings that you would normally throw away. Of course, you must scrub your potatoes well before peeling them.

SERVES 4

Scrubbed peelings from 4 potatoes

Freshly ground black pepper

Salt (optional)

1 Preheat the oven to 200°C/400°F/gas 6/fan oven 180°C.

2 Spread the potato peelings in a thin, even layer on a baking (cookie) sheet. Sprinkle with pepper and very lightly with salt, if liked.

3 Bake for about 20 minutes or until crisp and golden. Cool, then store in an airtight container.

Braised Cabbage with Celery, Apple and Walnuts

This is really good left to get cold, then reheated the next day. It can also be cooked in a saucepan over a fairly low heat, stirring occasionally. It is packed with energy-giving nutrients and is popular even with people who hate cabbage!

SERVES 4

---

450 g/1 lb red or white cabbage, shredded

1 onion, thinly sliced

2 celery sticks, chopped

1 cooking (tart) apple, chopped

50 g/2 oz/¹/₃ cup raisins

50 g/2 oz/¹/₂ cup chopped walnuts

30 ml/2 tbsp red or white wine vinegar

30 ml/2 tbsp water

30 ml/2 tbsp clear honey

Salt and freshly ground black pepper

15 g/¹/₂ oz/1 tbsp low-fat sunflower, soya or olive oil spread

30 ml/2 tbsp snipped fresh chives, for garnishing

---

1 Preheat the oven to 160°C/325°F/gas 3/fan oven 145°C.

2 Layer the cabbage, onion, celery, apple, raisins and walnuts in a casserole dish (Dutch oven).

3 Mix together all the remaining ingredients except the low-fat spread and pour over. Cut the spread into small flakes and scatter over the surface.

4 Cover and cook in the oven for 1¹/₂ hours until tender. Stir well, then sprinkle with snipped chives.

5 Serve hot or cold.

Curried Spring Greens
with Sultanas

This will tempt even those of you who loathe green leafy vegetables. It's great with any grilled meat, fish or poultry – or try adding cooked leftover chicken to it and serving it with rice for a complete revitalising meal.

SERVES 4

---

450 g/1 lb spring (collard) greens, shredded

450 ml/³/₄ pt/2 cups vegetable or chicken stock, made with 1 stock cube

25 g/1 oz/2 tbsp low-fat sunflower, soya or olive oil spread

50 g/2 oz/¹/₃ cup sultanas (golden raisins)

10 ml/2 tsp curry paste

15 ml/1 tbsp lemon juice

Salt and freshly ground black pepper

45 ml/3 tbsp desiccated (shredded) coconut

1 Cook the spring greens in the stock in a large flameproof casserole dish (Dutch oven) for 3–5 minutes until just tender. Drain in a colander over a bowl to reserve the stock.

2 Melt the spread in the same pan and stir in the sultanas, paste and lemon juice. Add the reserved stock. Bring to the boil and boil rapidly, stirring until reduced by half and slightly thickened.

3 Return the greens to the pan, toss and season to taste.

4 Put the coconut in a non-stick frying pan (skillet) and heat, stirring all the time, until the coconut turns a golden brown. Sprinkle over the cooked greens.

5 Serve hot.

Broccoli and Tomato Cheese

Full of folate, vitamins A and C and phosphorus, this side dish makes a tasty, nutritious lunch if you serve it with some wholemeal bread rolls or chunks of crusty granary bread. As a side dish, you can enjoy it with any meat, poultry or fish, especially grilled meats.

SERVES 4

1 large head of broccoli

25 g/1 oz/¼ cup wholemeal flour

450 ml/¾ pt/2 cups milk

A knob of low-fat sunflower, soya or olive oil spread

5 ml/1 tsp made English mustard

75 g/3 oz/¾ cup grated low-fat Cheddar cheese

Salt and freshly ground black pepper

1 × 400 g/14 oz/large can of chopped tomatoes

15 ml/1 tbsp tomato purée (paste)

25 g/1 oz/½ cup bran flakes, crushed

1 Cut the broccoli into small florets. Cook in boiling, lightly salted water for 4–5 minutes until just tender. Drain and place in an ovenproof serving dish.

2 Preheat the oven to 190°C/375°F/gas 5/fan oven 170°C. Whisk the flour with the milk in a saucepan until smooth. Add the low-fat spread. Bring to the boil and cook for 2 minutes, stirring, until thickened and smooth.

3 Stir in the mustard, 50 g/2 oz/½ cup of the cheese and salt and pepper to taste.

4 Mix the tomatoes with the tomato purée and spoon over the broccoli. Cover with the cheese sauce.

5 Scatter the remaining cheese and the bran flakes over.

6 Bake in the oven for about 35 minutes until golden and bubbling. Serve hot.

Stir-fried Point Cabbage with Sesame Seeds

Stir-frying cabbage means it is quickly cooked so preserves nearly all its nutrients. It tastes wonderful with nutty sesame seeds, which add B-vitamins and fibre to the dish. It is perfect with lean grilled pork chops, but it also goes very well with chicken or beef.

SERVES 4

30 ml/2 tbsp sunflower oil

5 ml/1 tsp sesame oil

1 small point cabbage, shredded

1 bunch of spring onions (scallions), cut into short lengths

1 garlic clove, crushed

45 ml/3 tbsp sesame seeds

Salt and freshly ground black pepper

1 Heat the oils in a wok or large frying pan (skillet). Add the cabbage and spring onions and stir-fry for 4 minutes.

2 Add the garlic and the sesame seeds and sprinkle with a pinch of salt and lots of pepper. Toss for 1 further minute.

3 Serve very hot.

Roasted Mediterranean Vegetables with Rosemary and Pine Nuts

Roast vegetables may not be original but they're absolutely a must on any fatigue-fighting diet plan. All those peppers supply loads of vitamin C and the pine nuts add a touch of B-vitamins and phosphorus too. Enjoy them with any grilled meat, fish or poultry or on their own, either hot, or cold as a salad.

SERVES 4

2 red (bell) pepper, cut into quarters

1 green pepper, cut into quarters

1 yellow pepper, cut into quarters

1 large courgette (zucchini), cut diagonally into slices

1 aubergine (eggplant), cut into slices

2 red onions, each cut into 6 wedges

30 ml/2 tbsp olive oil

2 small sprigs of fresh rosemary

50 g/2 oz/¹/₂ cup pine nuts

1 Preheat the oven to 200°C/400°F/gas 6/fan oven 180°C. Spread all the prepared vegetables in a large, shallow baking tin (pan). Drizzle with the olive oil and toss with your hands to coat completely.

2 Lay the sprigs of rosemary on top and sprinkle with the pine nuts.

3 Bake in the oven for 45 minutes, turning once or twice, until tender and slightly charred round the edges.

4 Discard the rosemary before serving hot or cold.

Creamy Flageolets with Garlic

The glorious, creamy texture of flageolets blends beautifully with garlic and crème fraîche to make a delicious accompaniment to meat or poultry. Make sure you always serve a green or orange vegetable too or a green salad, to get the best combination of revitalising nutrients.

SERVES 4–6

2 × 350 g/12 oz/medium cans of flageolet beans

1 garlic clove, crushed

45 ml/3 tbsp low-fat crème fraîche

Salt and freshly ground black pepper

1 Drain and rinse the beans.

2 Place in a saucepan with the garlic, crème fraîche, a pinch of salt and lots of black pepper.

3 Toss over a gentle heat until piping hot.

Caraway Potatoes

This is a vitalising version of roast potatoes. You can cook these for a slightly shorter time in a hotter oven if that suits what else you are cooking.

SERVES 4

700 g/1½ lb potatoes, scrubbed and cut into large chunks

30 ml/2 tbsp sunflower oil

30 ml/2 tbsp caraway seeds

1 Preheat the oven to 180°C/350°F/gas 4/fan oven 160°C.

2 Tip the potatoes in a roasting tin (pan). Add the oil and toss with your hands to coat. Sprinkle with the seeds.

3 Roast towards the top of the oven for 1–1½ hours, turning once during cooking, until golden and tender.

Vegetables Vichy

This is a famous way of serving carrots but is even better when mixed with sweet potato and orange peppers too. This adds more of the energy-boosting nutrients you need with every meal.

SERVES 4

---

2 large carrots, cut into chunky pieces

1 sweet potato, diced

1 orange (bell) pepper, diced

450 ml/³/₄ pt/2 cups water

A pinch of salt

5 ml/1 tsp clear honey

15 g/¹/₂ oz/1 tbsp low-fat sunflower, soya or olive oil spread

Freshly ground black pepper

30 ml/2 tbsp chopped fresh parsley

1 Place all the vegetables in a flameproof casserole (Dutch oven) with the water, salt, honey and the low-fat spread.

2 Bring to the boil over a high heat.

3 Turn down the heat to fairly low. Simmer, uncovered, for 30 minutes, stirring occasionally, until the vegetables are tender and all the liquid has evaporated.

4 Add a good grinding of pepper and sprinkle with the parsley before serving.

DOZE-FREE DESSERTS

Some of these are high in starchy carbohydrates for slow-release energy, others are fresh and fruity to help give you all the vital vitamins and minerals – as well as carbohydrates in the form of natural sugars – that will help keep you bright-eyed and bushy-tailed.

I prefer to use honey as a sweetener, because of its health-giving properties, but just occasionally artificial sweetener granules are a useful alternative.

Fruit and Nut Baked Apples

An apple a day is supposed to keep the doctor away and it will help keep you awake too – especially when packed with nutritious dried fruits and nuts with just a dash of honey for a little extra sweetness. Best of all, these are simplicity itself to prepare.

SERVES 4

4 even-sized cooking (tart) apples

60 ml/4 tbsp dried mixed fruit (fruit cake mix)

30 ml/2 tbsp chopped mixed nuts

20 ml/4 tsp clear honey

1 Preheat the oven to 180°C/350°F/gas 4/fan oven 160°C.

2 Cut the cores out of the apples but leave them whole. Using a sharp knife, cut a line round the circumference of the apples, just cutting through the skin (this will prevent them bursting during cooking).

3 Place them in a baking tin (pan) and add about 5 mm/¼ in water to the tin.

4 Mix the fruit and nuts together and pack into the apples. Spoon a teaspoon of honey over each.

5 Bake in the oven for about 50 minutes to 1 hour until just tender.

6 Serve in individual dishes with the juices spooned over.

Rich Bread Pudding

This has many vital ingredients – slow-release carbohydrates, high-energy fruits, energy-converting B-vitamins and lots of fibre. It is also delicious served cold.

SERVES 6–8

100 g/4 oz wholemeal bread, cubed

150 ml/¹/₄ pt/²/₃ cup milk

3 eggs

60 ml/4 tbsp clear honey

5 ml/1 tsp ground cinnamon

5 ml/1 tsp mixed (apple-pie) spice

5 ml/1 tsp ground mace

175 g/6 oz/1 cup dried mixed fruit (fruit cake mix)

20 g/³/₄ oz/1¹/₂ tbsp low-fat sunflower, soya or olive oil spread, melted

2.5 ml/¹/₂ tsp artificial sweetener granules, for dusting (optional)

1 Put the bread in a bowl.

2 Add the milk and leave to soak for 30 minutes. Stir briskly with a fork until well broken up.

3 Preheat the oven to 180°C/350°F/gas 4/fan oven 160°C.

4 Lightly beat the eggs and mix in with the honey, spices and fruit. Brush a 1.25 litre/2¹/₂ pt/6 cup ovenproof dish with some of the low-fat spread.

5 Turn the mixture into the dish and level the surface. Trickle the remaining spread over the surface.

6 Bake in the oven for about 1 hour or until golden brown and set.

7 Cool slightly and dust with the sweetener, if liked.

8 Serve cut into pieces.

Blueberry, Apple and Almond Crumble

Packed with vitamins and minerals, this dessert won't sap your strength. I enjoy it with a spoonful of Greek-style plain low-fat or fat-free yoghurt. Don't go for sweet, sugary custard though or you'll undo all your good work!

SERVES 4

---

175 g/6 oz blueberries

3 green eating (dessert) apples, peeled, cored and thinly sliced

90 ml/6 tbsp clear honey

10 ml/2 tsp lemon juice

75 g/3 oz/³⁄₄ cup ground almonds

75 g/3 oz/1¹⁄₂ cups fresh wholemeal breadcrumbs

2.5 ml/¹⁄₂ tsp ground cinnamon

50 g/2 oz/¹⁄₄ cup low-fat sunflower, soya or olive oil spread

30 ml/2 tbsp flaked (slivered) almonds

1 Preheat the oven to 180°C/350°F/gas 4/fan oven 160°C.

2 Place the blueberries and apples in a shallow, ovenproof dish with half of the honey and the lemon juice.

3 Mix together the ground almonds, breadcrumbs and cinnamon.

4 Melt the low-fat spread with the remaining honey. Stir into the crumble mixture until well blended.

5 Sprinkle the crumble mixture over the fruit and press down lightly.

6 Bake in the oven for 30 minutes, then remove from the oven and sprinkle the flaked almonds over the top.

7 Bake for a further 15–20 minutes until golden brown on top.

Apple and Sultana Strudel

Filo pastry is low in fat so great for fatigue fighters!
Here it is made into parcels of apples and sultanas – both
energy-boosting ingredients.

SERVES 4–6

2 cooking (tart) apples, peeled, cored and thinly sliced

45 ml/3 tbsp clear honey

2.5 ml/½ tsp ground cinnamon

Finely grated zest of ½ lemon

45 ml/3 tbsp sultanas (golden raisins)

4 sheets of filo pastry (paste)

15 g/½ oz/1 tbsp low-fat sunflower, soya or olive oil spread, melted

5 ml/1 tsp artificial sweetener granules

1 Preheat the oven to 190°C/375°F/gas 5/fan oven 170°C.

2 Mix the apples with the honey, cinnamon, lemon zest and sultanas.

3 Lay a sheet of filo on a clean cloth or piece of greaseproof (waxed) paper and brush very lightly with low-fat spread. Lay a second sheet on top and brush again. Repeat with the remaining two sheets, so you have a stack of four.

4 Spoon the apple mixture along the length of the pastry, just in from the edge.

5 Using the cloth or paper to help, roll the pastry over the filling to form a sausage shape.

6 Brush a baking (cookie) sheet with some of the remaining spread. Carefully lift the strudel and place on the sheet in a horseshoe shape.

7 Brush with any remaining spread. Bake in the oven for about 20–25 minutes or until the pastry is golden and the apple is cooked.

8 Sprinkle the sweetener over the surface. Serve warm.

Cinnamon Poached Pears

You've probably often seen recipes for pears poached in red wine. Here I use grape juice, which gives a lovely light flavour. There is nothing wrong with using wine – the alcohol is evaporated in the cooking – but the grape juice gives you the sweetness you need without the need for extra sugar.

SERVES 4

---

15 ml/1 tbsp clear honey

5 ml/1 tsp lemon juice

5 cm/2 in piece of cinnamon stick

300 ml/¹/₂ pt/1¹/₄ cups red pure grape juice

4 pears, peeled

1 Preheat the oven to 160°C/325°F/gas 3/fan oven 145°C.

2 Put the honey, lemon juice, cinnamon and grape juice in a saucepan and bring to the boil.

3 Cut a thin slice off the bottom of each pear so it will stand upright, and gently cut out the cores with a sharp, pointed knife.

4 Lay the pears in an ovenproof dish and pour over the juice mixture. Cover with foil and bake in the oven for 30 minutes, turning once. Remove the cinnamon stick.

5 Stand each pear in a dessert bowl and spoon the juice over. Serve hot or chilled.

Baked Peach and Almond Brûlée

This one is great for a dinner party! Elegant and delicious, but still packed with vitality: what more could you ask for?

SERVES 4

1 × 425 g/15 oz/large can of peach slices in natural juice, drained, reserving the juice

10 ml/2 tsp cornflour (cornstarch)

5 ml/1 tsp lemon juice

150 ml/¼ pt/⅔ cup plain low-fat yoghurt

1 large egg

2.5 ml/½ tsp ground mixed (apple-pie) spice

45 ml/3 tbsp clear honey

45 ml/3 tbsp flaked (slivered) almonds

1 Preheat the oven to 180°C/350°F/gas 4/fan oven 160°C.

2 Put the peaches in a 900 ml/1½ pt/3¾ cup ovenproof dish.

3 Using a wire whisk, mix the cornflour with a little of the reserved juice in a saucepan. Stir in the remaining peach juice and the lemon juice. Bring to the boil, stirring until thickened and clear. Allow to bubble for 1 minute, then pour over the peaches.

4 Whisk the yoghurt with the egg and spice. Pour over the peaches.

5 Bake in the oven for about 20 minutes until the custard is set.

6 Preheat the grill (broiler). Mix the honey with the almonds and spoon over the top of the pudding. Place under the grill until the honey bubbles and the nuts are golden. Remove from the grill immediately so the nuts don't burn.

7 Serve warm.

Fresh Mixed Citrus Jelly with Crushed Grapefruit

This is taste-tingling and delicious. It clears the palate and refreshes the most tired and listless body, leaving you feeling ready for anything.

SERVES 4

Finely grated zest and juice of 1 orange

Finely grated zest and juice of 1 lemon

15 ml/1 tbsp powdered gelatine

1 × 410 g/14¹/₂ oz/large can of grapefruit segments in natural juice

About 300–450 ml/¹/₂–³/₄ pt/1¹/₄–2 cups pure orange juice

1 Put the orange and lemon zests and juices in a measuring jug and sprinkle the gelatine over. Leave to soften for 5 minutes.

2 Stand the jug in a pan of hot water and stir until the gelatine has dissolved. Alternatively, heat briefly in the microwave.

3 Drain the grapefruit segments, reserving the juice, and pour the juice into the gelatine mixture. Make up to 600 ml/1 pt/2¹/₂ cups with pure orange juice.

4 Crush the grapefruit segments, discarding any membranes. Place in an attractive glass serving dish and pour in the juice mixture. Stir well. Chill until set.

Winter Fruit Compôte with Lime Cheese

The dried fruit salad is deliciously sweet as well as being packed with fatigue-fighting nutrients. Served with a zesty lime cheese, it makes the perfect end to a meal.

SERVES 4–6

225 g/8 oz/1½ cups dried fruit salad

50 g/2 oz/⅓ cup dried cranberries

50 g/2 oz/⅓ cup dried blueberries

300 ml/½ pt/1¼ cups water

300 ml/1½ pt/1¼ cups pure apple juice

Finely grated zest and juice of 1 orange

For the cheese:

200 g/7 oz/scant 1 cup low-fat soft cheese

Finely grated zest of 1 lime

10 ml/2 tsp clear honey

60 ml/4 tbsp low-fat crème fraîche

1 Put all the fruits in a saucepan with the water, the apple juice and the orange zest and juice. Bring to the boil, reduce the heat, part-cover and simmer very gently for 20 minutes. Remove from the heat and leave to cool.

2 Drain off any whey from the cheese, then stir in the lime zest and honey. Lastly, fold in the crème fraîche. Chill to firm slightly.

3 Spoon the fruits into shallow bowls and top each with a spoonful of the lime cheese.

Tropical Fruit Salad

Exotic fruits, simply prepared in apple juice with just a dash of honey for sweetness, make a great vitality-inducing dessert for any special occasion. For speed, you can use a 350 g/ 12 oz/large can of pineapple chunks in natural juice, rather than a fresh pineapple, if you prefer.

SERVES 4–6

300 ml/½ pt/1¼ cups pure apple juice

15 ml/1 tbsp clear honey

2 pomegranates

1 passion fruit

2 oranges

1 mango

2 kiwi fruit

1 small pineapple

Sprigs of mint, for decorating

1 Put the apple juice in a large plastic container with a lid and stir in the honey.

2 Halve the pomegranates and passion fruit and squeeze out the juice (as you would for a lemon). Strain the juice into the apple juice and honey mixture.

3 Hold the oranges over the container (to catch any juice) and cut off all the rind and pith, then slice and halve the slices.

4 Peel the mango and cut all the flesh off the stone (pit) in long strips. Halve the strips if very large.

5 Peel and slice the kiwi fruit. Cut all the skin off the pineapple, slice the fruit, then cut into chunks, discarding any thick, central core.

6 Add all the prepared fruit to the container. Stir gently to mix, then chill.

7 Serve in glass dishes, decorated with tiny sprigs of mint.

Summer Pudding

Slow-release carbohydrates and quick-boost energy are combined in this delicious recipe. Raspberries, blackberries, blackcurrants and strawberries all work well in this, but if you are short of berry fruits, add some peeled, cored and thinly sliced green eating apple to the mix.

SERVES 6

900 g/2 lb soft fruit, sliced or quartered if large

60 ml/4 tbsp water

About 30 ml/2 tbsp clear honey

8 slices of wholemeal bread, crusts removed

1 Put the fruit in a saucepan with the water.

2 Heat gently until the juices run and the fruit is soft but still holding its shape. Sweeten to taste with honey, adding just a little at a time.

3 Line a large pudding basin with about six slices of the bread, cutting to fit.

4 Spoon in the fruit and juice, reserving a spoonful of juice (you will need this to moisten any dry bread still visible when the dish is ready to serve). Cover with the remaining bread, again trimming to fit and filling in any gaps.

5 Stand the basin on a small plate and cover with a saucer or small plate. Top with weights or a couple of cans. Chill overnight.

6 When ready to serve, loosen the edge of the pudding with a round-bladed knife. Turn out on to a shallow serving dish. Use the reserved juice to 'touch up' any dry bread not soaked in juice.

7 Serve cut into wedges.

Chilled Light Lemon Cheesecake

I had planned to use sugar-free jelly for this recipe but couldn't get a lemon-flavoured one anywhere. Then I had this brainwave of using sugar-free squash – and it worked beautifully. Use a good-quality one with real lemons for the best taste and nutritional value. It makes a delicious, light pudding that won't make you nod off!

SERVES 6–8

200 ml/7 fl oz/scant 1 cup water

1 sachet of powdered gelatine

100 ml/3½ fl oz/scant ½ cup sugar-free lemon squash cordial

200 g/7 oz/scant 1 cup low-fat soft cheese

15 ml/1 tbsp clear honey

175 g/6 oz/1½ cups crushed digestive biscuits (graham crackers)

75 g/3 oz/⅓ cup low-fat sunflower, soya or olive oil spread, melted

150 ml/¼ pt/⅔ cup low-fat crème fraîche

Ground cinnamon, for dusting

1 Put 60 ml/4 tbsp of the water in a small bowl. Sprinkle the gelatine over and leave to soften for 5 minutes. Stand the bowl in a pan of simmering water and stir until the gelatine has completely dissolved. Alternatively, heat briefly in the microwave but do not allow to boil.

2 Stir in the remaining water and the lemon cordial, then whisk in the cheese and honey. Chill until the consistency of egg white.

3 Meanwhile, mix the crushed biscuits with the melted low-fat spread. Tip into a 20 cm/8 in flan tin (pie pan) and press down well to form a flan case (pie shell). Chill.

4 When the cheese mixture is on the point of setting, fold in the crème fraîche. Turn into the flan case and chill until set.

5 Decorate with a dusting of ground cinnamon before serving cut into wedges.

Creamy Rice Pudding

Rice for slow-release energy again – don't knock it, it's the best! Here I use low-fat evaporated milk for extra creaminess and flavour – it makes it taste more like canned Devon rice pudding, without any refined sugar.

SERVES 4

50 g/2 oz/¼ cup round-grain (pudding) rice

30 ml/2 tbsp clear honey

1 × 400 g/14 oz/large can of low-fat evaporated milk

A little grated nutmeg

1 Preheat the oven to 180°C/350°F/gas 4/fan oven 160°C.

2 Put the rice and honey in a 1.2 litre/2 pt/5 cup ovenproof serving dish.

3 Add the evaporated milk and stir until the honey dissolves.

4 Fill the can with water and add to the milk and rice, stirring until completely blended.

5 Dust the top with grated nutmeg.

6 Bake in the oven for about 1½ hours until golden on top. The rice should be tender and creamy.

7 Serve hot.

Almond Jelly
with Raspberry Coulis

This is cool, smooth and remarkably attractive to look at as well as being an energy-giving pudding, perfect for rounding off any elegant meal.

SERVES 4

For the jelly:

600 ml/1 pt/2½ cups milk

1 sachet of powdered gelatine

60 ml/4 tbsp clear honey

50 g/2 oz/½ cup ground almonds

2.5 ml/½ tsp natural almond essence (extract)

For the coulis:

225 g/8 oz raspberries

15 ml/1 tbsp lemon juice

4 tiny sprigs of mint

1 Make the jelly. Pour 90 ml/6 tbsp of the milk into a small bowl. Add the gelatine and leave to soften for 5 minutes. Stand the bowl in a pan of hot water or heat briefly in the microwave and stir until the gelatine is completely dissolved.

2 Stir this mixture into the remaining milk with 30 ml/ 2 tbsp of the honey, the ground almonds and the almond essence.

3 Pour into four lightly oiled ramekin dishes (custard cups). Leave to cool, then chill until set.

4 Meanwhile, reserve eight raspberries, then pass the remainder through a sieve (strainer) into a bowl and stir in the remaining honey and the lemon juice.

5 Carefully loosen the edges of the jellies and turn them out on to individual plates. Spoon a little raspberry coulis around and decorate each plate with two raspberries and a tiny sprig of mint.

Dashing Desserts in a Hurry

If you haven't got time – or the inclination – to cook fabulous desserts every day, here are a few quick and easy ideas that will keep you boosted, not bloated!

- Low-fat, 'diet' fruit yoghurt or fromage frais with a piece of matching or contrasting fruit, cut up, to dip in to it

- A banana, mashed and folded into a small tub of low-fat plain cottage cheese with a pinch of ground mixed (apple-pie) spice

- A wedge of melon, dusted with a little ground ginger

- Sugar-free jelly (jello) set with fruit, either fresh or canned in natural juice (if using canned, drain and use the juice as part of the liquid to make up the jelly)

- An apple, cored and sliced, with a small piece of Edam cheese

- Canned fruit in natural juice, topped with a small spoonful of low-fat crème fraîche

- An individual portion of Camembert – grill (broil) briefly until just melting, if you have time – and a handful of grapes or fresh blueberries.

FATIGUE-FIGHTING BAKERY

It's best to avoid ordinary biscuits (cookies) and cakes most of the time as they contain large amounts of added sugar and fat, which will almost certainly help to induce fatigue. This selection of slow-release energy bakes will not only sustain you but also make you feel on top of the world. If you can't resist a trip to the bakery counter, go for plain currant buns rather than greasy Danish pastries, and semi-sweet digestive biscuits (graham crackers) rather than sweet, fatty shortcakes. Fruit cake is much better for you than a chocolate fudge cake, too.

Read the labels on cereal bars. They may appear to be full of good things as they contain whole grains, seeds, nuts and dried fruit, but they are also often extremely high in added sugar. The home-made ones in this chapter will serve you much better!

High-fibre Oatcakes

Crisp and delicious, high in fibre and slow-release carbohydrates but great at lowering cholesterol too. Have these for breakfast, as a snack or with cheese to round off a meal.

MAKES 8

75 g/3 oz/³⁄₄ cup medium oatmeal, plus extra for dusting

15 ml/1 tbsp oat or wheat bran

A pinch of salt

1.5 ml/¹⁄₄ tsp bicarbonate of soda (baking soda)

15 g/¹⁄₂ oz/1 tbsp low-fat sunflower, soya or olive oil spread, melted

60–75 ml/4–5 tbsp hand-hot water

1 Mix the oatmeal, bran and salt together in a bowl.

2 Stir in the melted spread and water to form a firm dough.

3 Dust the work surface with a little oatmeal and roll out the dough to a 25 cm/10 in round. Cut into eight wedges.

4 Heat a non-stick frying pan (skillet). Cook a few oatcakes at a time for about 3 minutes until firm. Turn over very carefully (so as not to break them) and cook for a further 2–3 minutes.

5 Cool on a wire rack. Store in an airtight container.

Fruit and Fibre Scones

Obviously high in fibre, these delicious scones are best served warm with just a scraping of low-fat sunflower, soya or olive oil spread. Don't have too much, though, or the added fat could make you feel a bit weary!

MAKES 6

100 g/4 oz/1 cup self-raising (self-rising) flour

100 g/4 oz/1 cup self-raising wholemeal flour

10 ml/2 tsp baking powder

50 g/2 oz/¼ cup low-fat sunflower, soya or olive oil spread

40 g/1½ oz/¼ cup raisins

40 g/1½ oz/¼ cup ready-to-eat dried apricots, chopped

About 120 ml/4 fl oz/½ cup buttermilk

To serve:

Low-fat sunflower, soya or olive oil spread

1   Preheat the oven to 220°C/425°F/gas 7/fan oven 200°C.

2   Mix the flours and baking powder in a bowl. Rub in the fat, then stir in the fruit.

3   Mix with the buttermilk to form a soft but not sticky dough.

4   Knead gently on a lightly floured work surface and pat out to a round about 2 cm/¾ in thick. Cut into six scones (biscuits), re-kneading and shaping the trimmings as necessary.

5   Place on a non-stick baking (cookie) sheet. Bake in the oven for about 15 minutes until they are risen and golden and the bases sound hollow when tapped.

6   Serve warm or cold, split, with a scraping of low-fat spread.

Granary and Sesame Seed Bread Sticks

These are great to nibble with drinks as well as served with meals. They are higher in fibre than bought bread sticks and much more tasty! They are a good snack when you need a slow-release energy top-up.

MAKES 24

300 ml/½ pt/1¼ cups milk

15 ml/1 tbsp olive oil

400 g/14 oz/3½ cups granary flour

50 g/2 oz/½ cup sesame seeds

A good pinch of salt

5 ml/1 tsp clear honey

10 ml/2 tsp easy-blend dried yeast

1 Warm the milk and oil in a saucepan or in a bowl in the microwave until hand-hot.

2 Add the remaining ingredients and mix to form a soft but not sticky dough.

3 Knead on a lightly floured surface for 5 minutes until smooth and elastic. Alternatively, place all the ingredients in a food processor and run the machine for 1 minute.

4 Place in an oiled plastic bag and leave in a warm place for about 45 minutes until doubled in bulk.

5 Preheat the oven to 220°C/425°F/gas 7/fan oven 200°C.

6 Knock back (punch down) the dough, then re-knead and cut into 24 equal pieces. Roll each into a thin sausage about 30 cm/12 in long.

7 Transfer the sticks to a non-stick baking (cookie) sheet. Bake in the oven for about 30 minutes until golden and crisp.

8 Cool on a wire rack. Store in an airtight container.

Hazelnut Shortbread Fingers

You'd almost think these were packed with sugar but they're not – just loads of energy-giving ingredients. I do like them dusted with just 2.5 ml/½ tsp caster sugar but, ideally, you should use artificial sweetener granules instead.

MAKES 18

100 g/4 oz/½ cup low-fat sunflower, soya or olive oil spread

75 g/3 oz/⅓ cup thick honey

1.5 ml/¼ tsp vanilla essence (extract)

75 g/3 oz/¾ cup plain (all-purpose) wholemeal flour

75 g/3 oz/¾ cup plain flour

75 g/3 oz/¾ cup ground hazelnuts (filberts)

1 Dampen an 18 × 28 cm/7 × 11 in Swiss roll tin (jelly roll pan). Line with non-stick baking parchment. Preheat the oven to 160°C/325°F/gas 3/fan oven 145°C.

2 Beat the low-fat spread, honey and vanilla essence together until light and fluffy.

3 Work in the flours and nuts until the mixture forms a soft dough.

4 Press the dough into the prepared tin and prick all over with a fork.

5 Bake in the oven for about 40 minutes until a pale golden brown.

6 Mark into fingers with a knife, then leave to cool in the tin.

7 Remove from the tin and store in an airtight container.

Banana and Pecan Tea Bread

This is lovely served with a scraping of low-fat soft cheese rather than low-fat spread. It is packed with nutrients, so makes a great energy-giving snack. It's also good toasted for breakfast.

MAKES 1 900 G/2 LB LOAF

2 large ripe bananas

5 ml/1 tsp bicarbonate of soda (baking soda)

45 ml/3 tbsp clear honey

1 large egg

50 g/2 oz/¼ cup low-fat sunflower, soya or olive oil spread

275 g/10 oz/2½ cups self-raising (self-rising) wholemeal flour

5 ml/1 tsp mixed (apple-pie) spice

50 g/2 oz/½ cup pecan nuts, finely chopped

1 Dampen a 900 g/2 lb loaf tin (pan) and line with non-stick baking parchment. Preheat the oven to 180°C/350°F/gas 4/fan oven 160°C.

2 Blend the bananas, bicarbonate of soda and honey briefly in a food processor (or mash thoroughly).

3 Add the egg and fat and blend in the processor (or beat with a wooden spoon) until smooth.

4 Add the flour and spice and blend briefly (or fold in) until mixed, then stir in the pecans.

5 Turn into the prepared tin and level the surface. Bake for about 50 minutes to 1 hour until risen, brown and firm to the touch.

6 Cool slightly, then turn out on to a wire rack, remove the paper and leave until completely cold. Serve sliced.

Spiced Winter Fruits Cake

Dried fruits are a great source of B-vitamins and are also good for a quick energy boost. When made into a cake with wholemeal flour, they make a perfectly balanced snack.

MAKES 1 CAKE

100 g/4 oz/½ cup low-fat sunflower, soya or olive oil spread

175 g/6 oz/¾ cup clear honey

120 ml/4 fl oz/½ cup pure pineapple juice

75 ml/5 tbsp water

1 × 250 g/9 oz packet of dried fruit salad, chopped

5 ml/1 tsp bicarbonate of soda (baking soda)

5 ml/1 tsp ground cinnamon

5 ml/1 tsp mixed (apple-pie) spice

225 g/8 oz/2 cups self-raising (self-rising) wholemeal flour

5 ml/1 tsp baking powder

1 large egg, beaten

30 ml/2 tbsp milk

1 Dampen a deep 20 cm/8 in round cake tin (pan) and line with non-stick baking parchment. Preheat the oven to 180°C/350°F/gas 4/fan oven 160°C.

2 Put all the ingredients except the flour, baking powder, egg and milk in a saucepan and bring to the boil. Boil for 1 minute, then remove from the heat. Leave to cool for 5 minutes.

3 Stir in the remaining ingredients, turn the mixture into the prepared cake tin and level the surface.

4 Bake in the oven for about 1 hour 10 minutes or until it is a deep golden brown and a skewer inserted in the centre comes out clean.

5 Cool in the tin for 10 minutes, then turn out on to a wire rack, remove the paper and leave until cold.

Mixed Fruit Flapjacks

I like using jumbo oats for this recipe but ordinary porridge oats will do just as well. They are both high in fibre and complex carbohydrates with extra vitamins and minerals for a really nutritious nibble that is great at lowering cholesterol.

MAKES 12

---

100 g/4 oz/¹/₂ cup low-fat sunflower, soya or olive oil spread

100 g/4 oz/¹/₂ cup thick honey

30 ml/2 tbsp clear honey

75 g/3 oz/¹/₃ cup dried mixed fruit (fruit cake mix)

175 g/6 oz/1¹/₂ cups rolled oats

1 Preheat the oven to 180°C/350°F/gas 4/fan oven 160°C. Dampen an 18 cm/7 in square baking tin (pan) and line with non-stick baking parchment.

2 Melt the low-fat spread and all the honey together in a saucepan. Stir in the fruit and oats.

3 Press into the prepared tin. Bake in the oven for 30 minutes.

4 Mark into pieces, then leave to cool in the tin before cutting into fingers.

5 Store in an airtight container.

Carrot and Pecan Cake
with Apple Cheese Frosting

*Make sure you use carrots canned in plain water, rather than
with salt and sugar added. The topping has no icing sugar so
is a brilliant energy-giving alternative to the more usual
sugar-laden iced cake.*

MAKES 1 CAKE

For the cake:

175 g/6 oz/³/₄ cup low-fat sunflower, soya or olive oil spread

175 g/6 oz/³/₄ cup thick honey

250 g/9 oz/2¹/₄ cups self-raising (self-rising) flour

5 ml/1 tsp baking powder

2 large eggs

1 × 300 g/11 oz/medium can of carrots, drained

2.5 ml/¹/₂ tsp mixed (apple-pie) spice

75 g/3 oz/³/₄ cup pecan nuts, chopped

For the frosting:

2 green eating (dessert) apples, peeled, cored and sliced

75 ml/5 tbsp water

5 ml/1 tsp powdered gelatine

75 g/3 oz/¹/₃ cup low-fat soft cheese

5 ml/1 tsp thick honey

A few pecan halves, for decorating

1 Preheat the oven to 180°C/350°F/gas 4/fan oven 160°C.
   Grease a 900 g/2 lb loaf tin (pan) and line the base with
   non-stick baking parchment or greased greaseproof
   (waxed) paper.

2 Put all the cake ingredients in a bowl and beat with a
   wooden spoon until well blended (or do this in a mixer
   or food processor).

3 Turn the mixture into the tin and level the surface. Bake in the oven for about 1 hour until risen and golden and the centre springs back when lightly pressed.

4 Cool slightly, then turn out on to a wire rack, remove the paper and leave until completely cold.

5 Meanwhile, make the frosting. Put the apples in a saucepan with the water. Cover and cook fairly gently until really soft and pulpy.

6 Stir in the gelatine until completely dissolved.

7 Beat in the cheese and honey until the mixture is fairly smooth. Leave until cool, then chill until set.

8 Spread the frosting over the top of the cold cake and decorate with a few pecan halves.

9 Store in an airtight container in the fridge.

Peanut Sweetmeal Snacks

These shouldn't be eaten too often as the biscuits in the recipe do contain some refined sugars – albeit far less than most. However, the peanuts are an excellent source of zinc, which rather makes up for that! These will definitely top-up the energy levels.

MAKES 12

---

50 g/2 oz/¼ cup low-fat sunflower, soya or olive oil spread

45 ml/3 tbsp thick honey

60 ml/4 tbsp unsalted crunchy peanut butter

Finely grated zest of 1 lime or 1 small lemon

225 g/8 oz/2 cups finely crushed digestive biscuits (graham crackers)

---

1 Dampen an 18 cm/7 in square shallow baking tin (pan) and line with non-stick baking parchment.

2 Melt the low-fat spread, honey and peanut butter together.

3 Stir in the zest and biscuit crumbs until thoroughly blended.

4 Press the mixture into the prepared tin and leave to cool, then chill until firm.

5 Cut into fingers and store in an airtight container.

Energy Boost Bars

Designed to be a better option than bought cereal bars, these are delicious and full of nutrition. If you do buy cereal bars, check the ingredients and choose ones high in fruit and nuts and low in added sugar.

MAKES 15

1 × 175 g/6 oz/small can of low-fat evaporated milk

75 g/3 oz/¹/₃ cup thick honey

45 ml/3 tbsp pure apple juice

175 g/6 oz/³/₄ block of coconut cream

100 g/4 oz/²/₃ cup sultanas (golden raisins)

225 g/8 oz/1¹/₄ cups ready-to-eat dried apricots, chopped

225 g/8 oz/2 cups rolled oats

1 Heat the milk with the honey, apple juice and coconut cream until the cream melts.

2 Stir in the sultanas, apricots and oats. Mix well.

3 Dampen and line an 18 × 28 cm/7 × 11 in Swiss roll tin (jelly roll pan).

4 Press the mixture into the tin, then leave until cool. Chill until firm.

5 Cut into bars and store in an airtight container in the fridge.

Date and Pistachio Squares

A cross between small cakes and biscuits, these squares are highly nutritious and totally delicious. You can use almonds instead of pistachios if you like and dried apricots or peaches are good instead of dates, too.

MAKES 16

175 g/6 oz/³⁄₄ cup low-fat sunflower, soya or olive oil spread

175 g/6 oz/³⁄₄ cup thick honey

100 g/4 oz/²⁄₃ cup chopped dates

A few drops of almond or vanilla essence (extract)

2 eggs, beaten

225 g/8 oz/2 cups plain (all-purpose) wholemeal flour

30 ml/2 tbsp baking powder

40 g/1¹⁄₂ oz/¹⁄₃ cup pistachio nuts, chopped

1 Preheat the oven to 180°C/350°F/gas 4/fan oven 160°C. Dampen and line an 18 × 28 cm/7 × 11 in shallow baking tin (pan) and line with non-stick baking parchment.

2 Melt the low-fat spread with the honey in a saucepan and stir in the dates. Cool slightly, then beat in the essence and eggs. Fold in the flour, baking powder and half the pistachios.

3 Turn into the prepared tin and level the surface. Sprinkle with the remaining pistachios and bake in the oven for about 30 minutes or until risen and golden and the centre springs back when lightly pressed.

4 Cool slightly, then cut into squares and cool on a wire rack.

Sustaining Snacks in a Hurry

Here are a few more ideas for fatigue-fighting snacks when you feel you need something to eat between meals. Remember, it's not a good idea to reach for the biscuit tin or a chocolate bar, as those will only give you a quick boost and then your energy levels will take a dive. Here are some healthier options.

- A piece of fresh fruit
- A currant bun (unbuttered)
- A plain digestive biscuit (graham cracker)
- A wholegrain crispbread with a scraping of Marmite or peanut butter
- A crisp cereal bar with a high fruit and nut content (avoid those that are chewy or coated in chocolate)
- A rice cake, topped with a little flavoured low-fat soft cheese
- A small handful of raw peanuts
- A small handful of ready-to-eat dried fruit, e.g. apricots, peaches, pears, prunes
- A small packet of sunflower or pumpkin seeds
- A small packet of nuts and raisins

NON-ALCOHOLIC DRINKS

Alcohol induces fatigue but it isn't much fun sipping mineral water all night. Here are some really delicious concoctions for you to try. If you can't bear to have no alcohol at all, simply have one or two of these, perhaps, instead of pre-dinner drinks at a party and then have a couple of glasses of wine with the meal. That way you should still feel lively by the end of the evening.

Banana Daiquiris

Don't overdo the rum essence or you'll get a nasty shock!

SERVES 4

1 ripe banana, broken into pieces

250 ml/8 fl oz/1 cup pure pineapple juice

1.5–2.5 ml/¼–½ tsp rum essence (extract)

5 ml/1 tsp ground ginger

Juice of 2 limes

15 ml/1 tbsp clear honey

Cracked ice

1 Put the banana in a blender or food processor with all the ingredients except the ice. Run the machine until smooth and thick.

2 Fill four tumblers with cracked ice and pour in the cocktail. Serve at once.

Black Watch

Make sure you use pure grape juice, not a grape juice drink as they are full of sugar.

MAKES 6 GLASSES

600 ml/1 pt/2½ cups pure red grape juice

30 ml/2 tbsp sugar-free real blackcurrant cordial

Crushed ice

Sparkling mineral water

1 Mix the juice and cordial together.

2 Fill tumblers with crushed ice. Pour in the juice mixture and top up with sparkling mineral water.

3 Stir with a swizzle stick and serve straight away.

Raspberry Refresher

Zippy and fruity, this is delicious, particularly in the summer.

MAKES 6 GLASSES

1 × 300 g/11 oz/medium can of raspberries in natural juice

600 ml/1 pt/2½ cups pure apple juice

300 ml/½ pt/1¼ cups pure pineapple juice

Ice cubes

Sparking mineral water

1 Put the raspberries and their juice in a blender with the pure fruit juices. Blend well.

2 Strain into tall glasses. Add ice cubes.

3 Top up to taste with naturally sparkling mineral water and stir with a swizzle stick.

Sparkling Melon Punch

Use a pack of frozen, melon balls thawed, if you prefer. Don't use canned ones though, as they are always packed in syrup.

SERVES 6–8
1 small honeydew melon
600 ml/1 pt/2½ cups pure apple juice
15 ml/1 tbsp clear honey
15 ml/1 tbsp lemon juice
20 fresh mint leaves
2 handfuls of ice cubes
600 ml/1 pt/2½ cups sugar-free ginger ale

1 Cut the melon in half and scrape out and discard the seeds. Scoop out the flesh into a blender.

2 Add the apple juice and honey and lemon juice. Blend until smooth, then chill.

3 When ready to serve, put ice cubes in tall glasses. Add a few mint leaves to each glass.

4 Pour over the melon mixture and top up with ginger ale. Stir and serve.

Papaya Sling

This is delicious on a warm summer's day.

SERVES 4
1 ripe papaya
15 ml/1 tbsp clear honey
2 limes
45 ml/3 tbsp low-fat crème fraîche
150 ml/¼ pt/⅔ cup semi-skimmed milk
Crushed ice

1 Peel the papaya, cut in half and remove the black seeds. Cut into pieces and place in a blender or food processor with the honey.

2 Squeeze the juice of one of the limes and add to the mixture with the crème fraîche and milk.

3 Run the machine until the mixture is thick and smooth.

4 Put crushed ice in glasses and pour the mixture over. Cut four slices off the remaining lime. Make a small cut into each from the centre to the edge and hang over the rim of each glass.

Mojito Mo

I had real mojitos on a recent holiday in Cuba. They were wonderful. I can't say this version is quite as good but as a non-alcoholic alternative it's fine!

SERVES 1

A small handful of fresh mint

1 lime or ½ lemon

10 ml/2 tsp clear honey

5 drops of rum essence (extract)

2 drops of peppermint essence

Crushed ice

Sparkling mineral water

1 Put the mint in a tall glass. Bruise well with a pestle or the end of a rolling pin.

2 Cut a slice off the lime or lemon for garnish, then squeeze the remainder and mix the juice with the honey, rum and peppermint essences. Add to the glass.

3 Fill with crushed ice and top up with sparkling mineral water. Stir well and serve.

Pear and Cinnamon Soda

A nutritious drink to make you forget there's no alcohol.

SERVES 4
---

1 × 410 g/14 oz/large can of pear quarters in juice

300 ml/½ pt/1¼ cups pure apple juice

5 ml/1 tsp ground cinnamon

60 ml/4 tbsp low-fat crème fraîche

8 ice cubes

Soda water

1 Put the pears and their juice, the apple juice, cinnamon and crème fraîche in a blender or food processor and run the machine until smooth and frothy.

2 Put the ice cubes in glasses. Pour over the pear mixture and top up with soda to taste. Stir again and serve.

Cuba Libre Libre

Well, a bit extreme maybe, but why not? The ginger gives the warmth, similar to the rum and the rum essence adds the flavour. Don't overdo the essence though, as it is very concentrated.

SERVES 1

Ice cubes

2 slices of lime

5 drops of rum essence (extract)

A pinch of ground ginger

Sugar-free cola

1 Fill a tall glass with ice cubes and add the lime slices, rum essence and ginger.

2 Top up with cola, stir well and serve.

T and G

All the flavour of a gin and tonic but no gin! I researched the ingredients that go into making gin and blended them together. The result is fun and surprisingly good!

SERVES 4–8

2.5 cm/1 in piece of fresh root ginger

1 stalk of lemon grass

10 ml/2 tsp juniper berries

5 ml/1 tsp coriander (cilantro) seeds

Thinly pared zest of ½ orange

Thinly pared zest of 1 lemon

1 cinnamon stick

2.5 ml/½ tsp freshly grated nutmeg

200 ml/7 fl oz/scant 1 cup boiling water

Ice cubes

Slices of lemon or lime

Sugar-free tonic water

1 Roughly crush the ginger, lemon grass, juniper berries and coriander seeds.

2 Tip into a clean, screw-topped jar and add the fruit zests, cinnamon stick, nutmeg and boiling water. Screw on the lid, shake well and leave until cold, then chill for at least 24 hours.

3 Strain the liquid and pour into four to eight tall glasses (depending on how strong you want the flavour). Add ice cubes and slices of lemon or lime.

4 Top up with sugar-free tonic, stir and serve.

Blackcurrant and Orange Mull

This is warming and soothing without being sleep-inducing. Great when the nights draw in.

SERVES 6

---

2 oranges

150 ml/¹/₄ pt/²/₃ cup sugar-free real blackcurrant cordial, undiluted

1 cinnamon stick

2 cloves

1 bottle of pure white grape juice

150 ml/¹/₄ pt/²/₃ cup water

1 Cut all the rind off the oranges and place in a saucepan. Squeeze the juice and pour through a fine sieve (strainer) into the pan.

2 Add the remaining ingredients. Heat gently, stirring, until very hot but not boiling.

3 Remove the orange rind and cinnamon stick and serve in glass mugs or thick glasses.

Red Mull

No, this is not a mis-spelling of a certain energy-boosting commercial drink. It is simply fruity, spicy and delicious.

SERVES 6

---

1 litre/1³/₄ pts/4¹/₄ cups red pure grape juice

300 ml/¹/₂ pt/1¹/₄ cups pure orange juice

1 lemon, sliced

1 orange, sliced

1 sachet of mulled wine spices

2.5 cm/1 in piece of fresh root ginger, crushed

1 Put all the ingredients in a pan.

2 Heat gently, stirring occasionally, until hot but not boiling. Squeeze the sachet of spices against the sides of the pan to extract maximum flavour.

3 Ladle into wine goblets and serve.

Christmas Spirit

This is based on a Swedish drink that is packed with alcohol. It's a 'light' version that doesn't lose out on any of the flavour.

SERVES 12

300 ml/¹/₂ pt/1¹/₄ cups pure apple juice

1 litre/1³/₄ pts/4¹/₄ cups pure white grape juice

75 g/3 oz/¹/₂ cup large stoned (pitted) raisins

15 ml/¹/₂ tbsp clear honey

2.5 ml/¹/₂ tsp almond essence (extract)

6 cardamom pods

2 cloves

5 cm/2 in piece of cinnamon stick

1 lemon, sliced

1 Put all the ingredients in a large pan.

2 Heat gently, stirring, until almost boiling. Turn down the heat as low as possible and leave the mixture to simmer for 20 minutes. Remove from the hob.

3 Ladle the liquid into small glasses and serve.

Light Coffee Float

A wonderful end to a meal. It's slightly indulgent because it does have some cream so, to avoid nodding off at the table, make sure you use a thick low-fat variety!

SERVES 1

5 ml/1 tsp clear honey

2.5 ml/¹/₂ tsp ground ginger

150 ml/¹/₄ pt/²/₃ cup very hot decaffeinated black coffee

30 ml/2 tbsp low-fat double (heavy) cream

1 Put the honey and ginger in a wine goblet. Stir with a metal spoon. Leave the spoon in the glass and pour in the hot coffee. Stir until the honey is dissolved.

2 Hold a cold spoon, rounded side up, over the coffee, with the tip of the spoon just touching the surface of the coffee. Slowly pour the cream over the spoon so it floats on top of the coffee.

Index